UNDER THE RED VELVET COVER

UNDER THE RED VELVET COVER

Conquering Victimhood and Breaking the Silence of Abuse,
Corruption and Family Secrets – My Life Journey

GRANT GARRIS

authorHOUSE®

AuthorHouse™
1663 Liberty Drive
Bloomington, IN 47403
www.authorhouse.com
Phone: 1-800-839-8640

© 2010 Grant Garris. All rights reserved.

No part of this book may be reproduced, stored in a retrieval system, or transmitted by any means without the written permission of the author.

First published by AuthorHouse 5/12/2010

ISBN: 978-1-4490-6912-4 (e)
ISBN: 978-1-4490-6910-0 (sc)
ISBN: 978-1-4490-6911-7 (hc)

Library of Congress Control Number: 2010906523

Printed in the United States of America
Bloomington, Indiana

This book is printed on acid-free paper.

Edited by Celene R. Pumphrey and LJW.

This book is dedicated to my partner Paul, for always believing in me and pushing me to follow my dreams; and to my two sons, who are my entire world and the reason this book came to be. Lastly, I dedicate this book to Nelly. Without her, this book and this life could not have been created.

My indisputable gratitude goes to all of the crusaders and pioneers who have stood up for equality and human rights, including Martin Luther King Jr., Maya Angelou, Harvey Milk, Matthew Shepherd and Rosa Parks. Some have lost their lives, and others still press forward, making our world more tolerant.

While this is a true story, I have changed some names. It is my story, and I've told it with sincerity. My great hope is that you, the reader, will find meaning in the message in a way that impacts your own life, and perhaps even in the life of a child.

CHAPTER I

GET OVER IT!

W hen the phone rang at the Selma Police Department, I felt exhilarated and frightened at the same time.

Today, I would learn the truth.

An efficient sounding female voice answered the phone, "Dallas County Police Department."

My heart was pounding in my throat, choking me. For a bizarre moment I feared I wouldn't be able to speak.

"Hello? Is anyone there?"

Where do I begin? What do I say? I need to know the truth, but I don't think I can speak.

I was a thirty-eight year-old successful executive standing in my high-rise office in Atlanta, feeling like I was about to reenter the gates of hell.

"Hello?" she said again, her voice slightly impatient now.

"Um, yes, I'm here. I have a quick question,"

"Yes sir, how can I help you?"

"I was needing . . . I mean I wanted to see . . . Well, what I need to know is . . ."

I took a deep breath to calm myself. An avid public speaker, I seldom run out of things to say.

"Yes ma'am, I need to speak with someone about a case that's twenty two years old."

"A case? What type of case?"

"A sexual abuse case."

"Here in Dallas County, sir?"

"Yes ma'am. It was about twenty-two years ago."

She said, "Let me transfer you."

Oh, great, she's going to transfer me to someone that's an expert at getting whack jobs off the phone. Why am I doing this? My family told me the results of the case years ago. Why was I questioning what they had told me all of these years?

A voice on the other end of the line interrupted my mental tirade.

"Records, this is Lucy."

Fidgeting with the phone cord and starting to sweat, as I tried to formulate the right type of sentence to tell her what I needed. I finally started "I'd like some information on a case that's about twenty-two years old," I said. My voice was shaky but getting firmer.

"Twenty two years ago, sir?" she said softly. "I don't know if I would even begin to know where to look for this information. We have archived all of that information and the files have been stored downstairs."

"Yes ma'am I understand that, but I was hoping to learn how the case ended," I replied. *This town was so corrupt back then and I just don't believe what I was told by my family is what happened. I honestly feel that he, at most, got a slap on the wrist. All of these years I have fooled myself into believing that in fact he did receive some type of criminal punishment.*

"Why do you need to know about this? Are you an attorney, sir?"

"No ma'am, I'm the person who filed the complaint." My voice cracked from nervousness as I tried my hardest not to sound petrified. *He was the one who did it to himself and I should have nothing to be ashamed of.*

Following a compulsion to tell her the truth, I hurried on, "Ma'am, I was a fifteen years old when I turned in my grandfather for sexually abusing me. I've heard so many stories about the verdict that I just wanted to verify the truth."

Now that I'd started, I couldn't stop.

"I've been trying to remember my childhood, and doing a lot of writing about my life and what I experienced at the hands of the devil known as my grandfather." Feeling I was losing her in my tumble of words, I finally paused and said, "I just need to know so I can move on."

She put me on hold for a while and came back on the line, her voice filled with quiet compassion. "Honey, it'll take me a couple of hours, but I'm going to go downstairs and try to find this for you. When did you report the abuse?"

I couldn't even remember what I had done last week, much less over twenty years ago regarding something I would rather forget. I knew I had to give her some type of additional information if I wanted to get anything out of this call.

"I don't remember the exact date, but I can tell you it was during the summer in the mid-eighties."

"Can you narrow it down a little bit for me? Everything we have is filed by date."

I was stunned into silence. There's so much of my childhood I can't remember. I was horrified I couldn't remember the exact date.

Holy shit, I'm going to have to call her back, and I don't know if I have the courage to make this phone call again. Think!

Remembering specifics about my past is like trying to remember where I put my car keys – *I know they have to be somewhere.* Desperate to recall the date, I searched my brain for clues. I couldn't tell her that the reason I was calling was to help *me* create a timeline of my life. There were huge chunks of my past missing, and I was working to fill in the blanks. These chunks were filled with darkness and unanswered questions because I had mentally blocked what was happening to me during that time. Like many young victims, I wiped out what was happening because it was too horrifying for a child's mind to comprehend.

Similar to walking around the house and retracing my steps to find my keys, I can run through events that help me recall elements from that darkness by identifying cultural or social events, even natural disasters. I can retrieve these events, but I can't remember what was happening to me during that time. Then it came to me.

"Wimbledon!"

She said, "Excuse me, sir,"

"Wimbledon had just been on television, and Boris Becker had won, so it must have been sometime in July 1985," I said, feeling my excitement growing as if I had just answered the last question on a tough college final exam correctly.

"Okay, let's try this, who was the perpetrator in the case?"

"My grandfather," I blurted, still reluctant to say his name.

She politely said, "Well, honey, I really need a name."

Why am I so compelled to know what happened? Should I just do what my cousin suggested and just "get over it?" No! I can't forget all of the past like that because it has, in some weird way, made me who I am today. I need to understand it more clearly. I need to know that all of the things I have done

3

have made some kind of a difference. I'm no longer a frightened teenager. I'm a man in search of my past and I knew the truth would literally set me free, or at least I hope.

"His name is Bernard Jowers," I said softly, speaking that wretched name aloud for the first time in years.

He is my mother's father and all of the grandchildren in the family called him Pop. We call my mother's mom Mema. They were thought to be the pillars of our family by friends and within their community.

Lucy put me on hold again while she searched for the grand jury verdict.

The lame elevator music on the other end of the line made my thoughts drift back to that bleak summer day when I finally told someone about Pop's dirty little secret.

Dad drove me to the courthouse and didn't say a word to me the entire ride.

I was hoping he would at least tell me things would be all right and that I was doing the right thing by going to the police. Instead, we sat in deafening silence. My desire to just get all of this behind me was palpable. I wondered if he would be proud of me for telling the details of what happened, or if he would be disgusted once he knew the truth about the horrible specifics I was getting prepared to tell.

My mind ran on, *Will this kill my relationship with everyone in my family or will it bring us closer together?*

I knew that regardless of the outcome, this was what I had to do for me.

As we rounded the corner and turned onto the road that led to the courthouse, I could feel my stomach start to churn with worry. I could feel my muscles trembling all over as if I were cold. We pulled into the parking lot and I took a deep breath. *It's too late to turn back now, I guess.*

I was terrified to relive all of the events that had happened to me because I had tried so hard to forget all about the gruesome details. The reality was that if I were going to find justice I would have to be forthcoming and honest about what had happened. I wanted him to go to jail forever just to keep him away from our family, and mostly from me. I was so angry because he put me in this situation where I, a teenager, had to do what I knew was right for both me and any other kids he could hurt.

Dad and I exited the car; the only sounds to be heard were the clinking of the keys as they were pulled out of the ignition and the release of the door as I pulled the handle. We greeted each other at the trunk of his car and he hesitantly put his arm on my shoulder. This was about as deep as his emotions could go, because he was trying to be supportive of me and still look like a man to everyone else.

"You OK?"

I was glad he'd finally spoken to me, but now was not the time for a conversation. I just wanted to be done with this.

"Yes, I'm fine, I guess."

I was standing beside him as we looked up the steps and the sun was glaring over the top of the historic building, blinding me briefly.

As I put my hand over my brow to block the sun, I could make out some people at the top of the steps. I couldn't tell exactly who they were but as we walked up the mountain of concrete steps I looked up at the wall of people and realized it was my family and friends who were there to support me, or so I thought.

Once we got closer, about six steps from the top, my Aunt Patricia greeted us and gently took my hand. For the first time that morning looking into Aunt Patricia's eyes, I felt safe and thought how wonderful it was they were all there to support me. As soon as our hands connected I could feel her confidence and power surround me almost like a body guard. For a short moment everything I feared and everything I was concerned about briefly went away as I became transfixed on her loving face.

With her other hand, she gently pulled my face close to hers. "Don't you worry about a thing, you are so wonderful and you are doing the right thing. I will be here for you all day if that is what you need. I am here for you in heart and soul. Do you understand me?"

Aunt Patricia was the wife of Uncle Nick, who was a Methodist preacher. She understood love better than anyone in our family and she had never gone back on her commitments to me.

Not really sure why she was telling me this, I knew she would not lie so I wanted to let her know that I trusted her immensely. "Aunt Patricia, I love you and I know you are here for me. Thank you so much for believing me."

As we finally reached the last foot of our climb and approached the other members of my family, I stepped forward to receive their words and their support. I discovered I couldn't have been more wrong about their presence. They were there to beg me not to talk to the police. They didn't want me to turn my grandfather in as a sexual predator.

I became frozen in my steps. I looked at all of them in disbelief, my mouth unable to move and my heart breaking with every word they uttered.

I started to tune them out and their words became distorted sounds that made no sense to me. My eyes went from one person to the other and I could feel my world shrinking by the second. I could feel the sweat start to bead up on my forehead and upper lip and I just wanted to take off running in any direction I could to get away from them.

It is breathtakingly easy to gang up on a child and to insert a seed of doubt in his mind. They did their best – after all, this was the family business; maintaining this façade was the sick and twisted glue that held them together. However, through all of this internal chaos, I was still confident about what I needed to do and held true to what I had discussed with my dear Nelly. *I had to do this for me because I was not the person that caused this and I am only doing the right thing.* This saying became my rote mantra to keep me focused.

Luckily, my mind-set took a turn in the proper direction. I became enraged at the audacity that any of these people would be here to support the person that had raped many of them, repeatedly, and continued to present a danger to their own children. At fifteen, I shouldn't be facing my family and doing something so difficult. They were all older and I can't believe it took me, the youngest person in the family, to finally say something about this monster. The tension and stress from the car ride quickly turned to anger. Finally, I silenced them with my words and started to reclaim the reason for me being there.

"This is something I have to do," I said angrily and loudly. "I have to stop him before he hurts any more kids."

"He won't hurt any more kids," my mom said, with a confidence she could not possibly feel. However, she was intent on her mission to silence me. She took a step down to get closer to me as my teen-aged mind tried to decide if she was there to support me or if she was there to protect her father. She continued, "At least, not kids outside our family." Question answered, and chillingly so.

I could feel the blood rush out of my face. *I thought she believed me. I thought she would be the one to support me all the way through this. I guess I am more alone than I thought.*

As she looked at me stoically, I stepped past her and reminded her about my two young cousins who lived next door to my grandparents. *Were they joking with me or were they serious? I couldn't believe that they were all quite aware that I was there to do the right thing, and yet they wanted me to stay silent as they had for so many years.* I was furious, and at that point more determined than ever. They were as sick as he was for trying to protect him. They were treating me as if I were turning in their cult leader.

My only concern was now removed. I was certain I would never have the same relationship with them and no longer did I care.

Without another word, my Aunt Patricia, with my hand in hers, gently pushed everyone aside as if she were completely dismissing them and endearingly pulled me into her body. She put her arm around me, protecting me as she calmly led me into the police station. She kissed me on top of my head and said, "Don't let the nonsense they are telling you change your mind. *You are doing the right thing and they are embarrassed that they didn't.*"

That sentence meant the world to me. I looked up into her bright green eyes and finally felt that someone understood what I was doing.

My parents eventually followed us inside. As we walked through the huge white doors that were framed with intricate hand carved molding, the brightness of the sun became gray. Inside, there were police officers scurrying around, walking from office to office. It smelled sterile and institutionalized like most government buildings. My aunt walked away briefly to find out where we needed to be and what we needed to be doing. Within minutes she had returned to guide us to a bench that was as old as the building.

"They said they would be right out," she told me.

As soon as we sat down on the bench a man approached us and asked if we were there to meet with a detective. My aunt stood, "Yes, that would be us."

She was speaking in the softest of tones but truly taking control of the entire situation. She was making sure that she knew what was going on and where we needed to be, keeping me informed along the way. She had appointed herself as my spokesperson and would not allow people to get in front of me without them explaining to her first what their expectations were from me. She was keeping her word and charging forward with supporting me.

We were led into an office where there was a desk, with two chairs that were covered with ugly green vinyl. They were strategically placed in front of an office desk facing the third larger chair positioned behind the desk. Prior to walking into the door of the office I imagined myself as a cat, not sure that I wanted to go into the room, with all four paws on each side of the door. Once I crossed the threshold I realized I had no reason to be intimidated by the room itself.

It was a makeshift office at best, without any phones and a window that overlooked the mountain of steps we had just climbed. I could hear the hum of the window unit air conditioner but I couldn't tell if it was cooling because of the adrenaline that surged through my body. The sound it made was soothing and drowned out the noise from the other offices. I was not sure if I should sit down or stand up so I just stood behind one of the chairs waiting on directions. The room felt so institutional and impersonal. I was doing everything I could to hold myself together and be strong. Part of me wanted to forget it all and the other part of me wanted to make sure I didn't leave out any details of what had taken place.

I turned back towards the doorway and saw two detectives, a man and a woman, walking toward us.

They must be the people to whom I'll have to tell my life-long dark secret.. I just hope they don't think I am lying. I just know once I tell them about this they will absolutely make sure that Pop will never see the outside of a jail cell. I am certain of that.

They came in and one sat behind the desk while the other one pulled up one of the green vinyl chairs. The man pointed to the other chair "Please have a seat."

As he looked at me, I slowly dropped down and sat on the edge of the seat. I looked over my left shoulder and saw Dad standing there and of course Aunt Patricia.

I scooted back into the chair and you could hear the squeak of the vinyl against my jeans.

The female detective slowly and carefully started with the questions. "So I understand that you have some information that you would like to share with us. I want you to know that you can completely trust us and we are here to keep you out of harm's way and to protect the other people who could possibly get hurt." I could feel the sincerity in her voice and I knew that regardless if they were sincere or not at this point it did not matter. I felt a light, cold sweat all over my body as I recalled everything I had recessed so far in the back of my mind. I told them how he came into my room at night, how he would stalk me throughout the house when he came home from work, how he'd taken me out on the boat where he knew I couldn't escape and physically tortured me when I tried to get away. I told them in great detail how he'd raped, brutalized, and abused me for his own sick pleasure throughout the past fifteen years.

When I finished, I was emotionally exhausted, but I felt as if I had finally started the process of getting justice for all of the pain this bastard had caused me.

The detectives took Dad and me to what they called a "holding room." It's funny but that strange room is one of my most vivid memories I can recall about the entire day. We were walking down a hallway between walls covered with wood paneling. I was surprised when one of the police officers just slid the wall open to reveal a room. It amazed me that they were able to create this secret location that was so invisible to the naked eye. Looking back it was ironic that this room was much like the abuse I had been through. It was hidden in plain sight and no one ever suspected it of being there. It was real and something that no one spoke of, because if it were discovered, it would have revealed the hiding place.

Though you couldn't see it from the hallway, it was huge. There was a little foyer that led to a larger room with two windows covered with bars. The floor was linoleum and the only items in the room were a sofa and a barstool with a phone on it. The room was a bit mustier smelling than the rest of the building, but as I got further into the room I realized why.

Dad asked, "Are you all right?"

By now, my generally taciturn father was at a complete loss for words. He had just heard, for the first time, the extent of abuse I had been through all of my life. He seemed shocked and was trying to stay strong, but his strength was silence.

"Yeah, I think so," I said. "Can I use the phone?"

I needed to get in touch with Mema before anyone else filled her head with lies.

"Sure," the police officer said.

I walked over to the brown and orange plaid sofa and sat down, and a cloud of dust arose around me. I had found the source of the odor. It was obvious this was not a room decorated for visitors and it was rarely used. The fabric on the couch felt like burlap to my forearms, but I didn't care because I was focused on the phone call I needed to make.

In front of the couch was a barstool with gray metal legs and a wooden seat. The phone was resting on top of it. I picked up the ugly beige phone and had to untangle the curly cord that had become tightly knotted from years of use.

Dad was off in the corner and we were wrapped in silence once again. I could tell he was still trying to process everything he had just heard. I was afraid he was ashamed of me so I didn't want to get engaged in a conversation. By reading his body language it was not obvious if he were disappointed that I had decided to stand up for myself, or embarrassed that I allowed myself to be abused. Either way I could not change what had happened.

I quickly dialed the phone number. I was so desperate to talk to her because I knew I'd probably never see her again. I was excited to finally tell her the truth about what had been happening all of these years. I thought I would be turning on a light in her life, revealing what a horrible monster her husband was.

She answered the phone on the first ring.

"Hi, Mema, it's me, Grant," I said.

I wanted to tell her that I just told the police what Pop has been doing to me and they're going to talk to him.

"What have you done this time?" she said viciously. "That's why Pop had to leave so quickly. I knew it had something to do with you."

I was speechless. Her tone had never been that harsh to me before. I knew she must have been told something that was not true.

Mema was a true Southern matriarch. It didn't take long to discover that she spoke softly but wielded great power. Disappointed and aware that now, more than ever, I was ostracized from my family; I was too hurt for tears. Realizing she wouldn't listen to anything I said, very timidly and softly I whispered, "I love you," and hung up.

I was despondent and certain I had done this to myself. My family was falling apart from every direction. I thought they would support me, but instead my world continued to just get smaller.

After I concluded the call, I stood up and glanced out the window. I saw Pop, the prominent citizen, Bernard Jowers, get out of his blue and white truck and retrieve something from inside his stainless steel tool box he had installed in the truck bed. I could see the sun reflect off of the lid as he was opening it and I was sure he was getting a gun.

I felt my tumultuous emotions from my phone call with Mema turn to fear and concern as I watched this six-foot four-inch man come charging toward the building

Pop is what Southern folks call a "good ole boy." He was entrenched in the local network and politics that controlled many aspects of life in our town, and had absolutely no fear of anything. As he walked out of my view, I thought my life would end soon because he was coming into the police station to start shooting everyone until he found me.

He had told me many, many times that if I told anyone what he had done he would kill me or my mom and that he didn't care about going to jail. I was absolutely terrified. I really felt he was going to come in and follow through on the threats he had petrified me with all my life.

My dad and I didn't talk as we sat in the strange hidden room. I was on one end of the couch with my hands buried between the couch seat cushion and the back of my thigh just staring into space and chewing on the inside of my cheek and lower lip. Dad sat at the other end of the couch and would shift his body from side to side.

Dad alternately sat back far into the couch and then close to the front edge of the cushion, unconsciously moving back and forth until he could no longer sit. He then stood up to pace. Then he would return back to the couch and start all over again. The silence was stifling. I couldn't breathe because of the panic I was feeling and the overpowering odor of mold in the room. I was terrified my grandfather was going to come through that secret door any moment.

It seemed like hours before the officer came back and told us it was safe to come out. I was hesitant to move because I knew Pop was still in the building.

The officer apparently understood the panic on my face so he explained to me what had just taken place. He said Pop had been arrested and was in jail. With a release of emotions, I fell into my dad's body and burst into tears, barely able to stand. I was physically and mentally fatigued. My nightmare was finally over, or so I thought.

Again my teenage logic was proven wrong. Only twenty-four hours later, Pop was out of jail, thanks to my uncle and his friends in the legal system.

The next day they all came to see me – my mom and Dad and Uncle Lance. I was asked if I thought it would be all right for Pop to be out of jail, "because someone needed to care for Mema," who was losing her sight due to a disease called retinitis pigmentosa. It caused the retina of her eyes to slowly deteriorate, eventually leading to full blindness.

"No," I said flatly. "It's not a good idea. If he gets out, he can go on hurting people and do to other kids what he did to me."

More than that, I feared even though he didn't kill me at the police station that didn't mean he wouldn't try – and succeed – somewhere else.

"You know that Mema is sick and someone needs to take care of her," Mom cloyingly said. "If he's in jail, then we'll have to move in with her." I was shocked that she was more concerned for this lady that harbored and protected his dirty little secret all of these years than she was for me, her own son.

11

"Why can't she come and live with us?" I was convinced it would be easier to upset her life than it would have been to stop what I had just started with the justice process.

"Because their home is the only place she knows how to walk around safely without hurting herself. If she came to live at our house, she'd have to learn how to get around all over again." This was a very weak argument to me but I felt out numbered.

I looked from one face to another – my father, my uncle, my mother – they were all trying to convince me to let the monster out of jail.

Didn't they understand what I had just been through? Didn't they know the effort it took to go against this entire family that was so tightly knit? I had to do something no one else had ever done. I was the youngest grandchild. Why hadn't one of these assholes done something to protect me from that bastard? Now they were asking me to ignore my efforts that had left me raw with exhaustion and let him out of jail.

I had no idea they were doing this to prevent me from knowing he was already out of jail.

All three of them looked at me as if I were a spoiled brat throwing a temper tantrum for not getting my way. My mom's expression made it clear I should just "get over it."

"He got out because he's going to get help," my mom said, her voice sounding smug to me. "He's going to see a doctor and get some therapy."

Feeling defeated, I responded the only way I knew how, with anger.

"I want proof. I want to see the papers that say he is seeing a doctor," I said. "As long as I know he's doing that, it will be all right."

I knew it would not be all right and I know they felt the same way. They went through the motions of accompanying me through all of this hell, reliving the abuse to strangers, just to appease me. She said OK with a hint of a smirk on her face.

That was the last I heard of it for the next twenty-one years.

There were no papers of any kind indicating he received counseling. I never heard anyone speak of Pop going to a psychiatrist nor did I hear them discuss anything about therapy. I was supposed to know about it, but once again, I had been consoled with a pack of lies.

Lucy's return to the phone line in Selma jerked me back to the present. "Mr. Garris, the verdict states there was not enough testimony or evidence to prosecute your grandfather, so the case was thrown out of court."

My body exploded with emotion. I felt stunned, shocked, and literally couldn't believe what I was hearing.

"What?" I yelled into the phone. "What do you mean, thrown out?"

Had everything I'd said been discarded like it was trash? Was I nothing but garbage? Did my testimony mean nothing? All of the things I told them about the abuse and torment I had gone through didn't matter?

With surprise in her tone, Lucy said, "You really didn't know this?"

I could tell by the change in the sound of her voice she was sincere, which helped to calm me.

"No I didn't. I was told that my uncle bailed him out of jail and that the courts ordered him to seek counseling or go to jail for life. I was told in lieu of serving time, he would get therapy. Is that not the case?"

I felt as if everything I wanted to believe all of these years was in fact distorted so I could feel as if I had been supported by them. After having Pop arrested, my family did give some lip service to being "proud of me for standing up to him" but the reality was they were all-too-willing to look the other way. I now knew that all of my fears were not fears at all, but instead the reality that my family would stand up for people who were sexual molesters over the children who were screaming out to help stop it. It was only thrown out because of their connections with other corrupt politicians and attorneys.

Lucy repeated that the case had been dismissed. Again, sounding very sympathetic she explained further, "Mr. Garris, give me some time. I'll go and pull the files on this case. You need to understand that I may not be able to get them today, because these cases usually have about 1,700 pages and are stored in boxes and multiple files. It's going to be a lot of stuff. Let me see what I can find, and I'll call you back."

I slowly lowered myself into my office chair and I turned and looked out at the view through my huge window on the fourteenth floor at the beautiful city that I now considered home. Struggling with being in the body of an adult and feeling like that same violated child I replied to her saying. "No problem," still trying to process all of it. "I live in Atlanta, Georgia, so please just let me know what you find. I can drive down there today if I have to, and pick the files up or at least copies of the files."

"I don't want you to have to do that, Mr. Garris, I can mail them to you," she said politely.

"Thanks, but I really have to see this for myself, and I need to know as soon as possible," I said, trying to convey my sense of urgency. "Do you think I should leave right now and just pick up the file when I get there?" I spun my chair around and broke my trance from looking at the amazing view. I saw that my car keys were where I always put them on the edge of my desk. I was grabbing for them when she stopped me.

"No sir. Let me see what I can find first. There really is no guarantee that I can even find the files from that long ago."

"Okay," I said reluctantly. "Thank you so much. I truly appreciate all your help because I'm so confused now. I just want to find out what happened."

I dropped the phone into its cradle, feeling I was cutting a vital connection. I really didn't want to hang up because I felt Lucy had the answers I'd been looking for most of my life. I feared by cutting off that connection I was losing what I needed to finish my story.

I sat at my desk unable to move and emotionless. Staring at the back of my closed office door, looking at my cable gym and its multi-colored cables I had hung up for working out while I was losing focus on conference calls, I realized that what I feared for years was true.

Still, I had a difficult time convincing myself the police would just "throw out the case" after everything I'd told them. The monster had raped me – repeatedly and violently. How could they just throw that out without talking to me first? Who gave the grand jury the right to throw out a case without letting the victim know? Naturally, if I had known anything about the criminal justice system at that time, I would have been aware that their failure to pursue my testimony was a signal that they were not actually investigating my case.

I was furious, hurt, confused, and just plain scared. I had to break my stare, so I stood up and paced in my office, back and forth like a caged animal, waiting for the phone to ring. I kept looking at the phone's display to be sure I had no missed calls. I checked the volume on the ringer to be sure it was loud enough to be heard easily.

I wanted to move, but I had to stay in place. I had to stay near the phone. My mind replayed my life like a series of video tapes. I could see the scared little boy, hiding in the house, doing everything possible to avoid the old man. No matter what I did, he had an uncanny ability to find me, just like a hunter sighting prey.

The scene moved to a scared little boy, trapped on a boat, with no place to go, no place to hide, feeling blood slowly drip down my leg from being raped, while burns throbbed from being thrown into the boat engine and reeking of gas.

Then I saw the frightened teenager walking up the courthouse steps, facing family and strangers telling them the horrors a child should never know.

Then I saw the determination I had throughout my life. I refused to give up my power and have this childhood affect my life and the image of the person I knew I could be despite all of the statistics.

Finally, after almost three hours, my phone rang. The number being displayed was Lucy calling. I answered in a professional manner, in case it was someone else from her office, but it was her friendly voice that greeted me.

"Hi, Mr. Garris. This is Lucy calling from Dallas County Records Division."

I felt my heart in my throat, and my pulse beating in my ears. At first I didn't know if I could even speak. I had been so desperate to learn about this, and now I wasn't sure I could tolerate the truth.

"Hello," I finally choked out. "I've been waiting for your call. Should I leave now so I can come and pick up the files?"

"No," she hesitated, "No, this entire file is very strange," she said quietly. "I've looked everywhere the files should be, and I can only find five pages of documents. I have to be honest with you, Mr. Garris. I have never found a file that went to the grand jury containing only five pages."

The tone of her voice indicated that she felt something wasn't quite right. She sounded almost as confused as I was. "Something must have happened to the file, but I really don't know what it could have been."

As soon as she said that, my biggest fears were confirmed. All the hope I'd carried that I would finally get answers was deflated. I knew immediately that Pop's and Uncle Lance's connections had made it happen. They had bribed their way out of the situation. This fear had been in the back of my mind for years, and now I had confirmed that the good ole boy network was stronger and thicker than blood.

Since the document was only five pages, Lucy promised to fax them right away.

As I sat there stunned, staring at my computer screen, waiting for the fax, I couldn't believe the sacrifice I had made had been for nothing. *Nothing.* The liars had won again.

I'd gone through my adult life believing I had done something honorable and right. In fact, however, I had poured out my heart and exposed one of the darkest secrets of my life to no avail.

The old man had won . . . again!

I sat at my desk, going through each encounter with my grandfather, remembering clearly each time I was abused, threatened, left crying and wounded, praying for death. I had shared all of it, and the case had been thrown out of court for 'lack of testimony.' Once again, the truth I told had been swept under the rug of lies my family protected like jewels in the family vault.

When the fax arrived, it took me several minutes to gain the courage I needed to read it. I think I was convincing myself if I didn't read it, I could still believe Pop had been punished and I'd gotten justice.

I knew if I did open it, I would realize that all of the effort and humiliation I put into turning Pop into the police had been for my families entertainment only.

All these years, I've been nothing but a fool to my entire family.

I slowly placed my finger on my mouse, closed my eyes, and double clicked, unwillingly opening the next chapter of my life.

CHAPTER 2

NELLY

Corruption and controversy are not new to Selma, Alabama. Frightening "Bloody Sunday", March 7, 1965, brought the Edmund Pettus Bridge right into America's living rooms. It was the day African Americans marched to get the right to vote without having to pass a test. To make it worse, it was a test most people could not have passed, regardless of their race. African Americans with Ph.D.s couldn't pass the test, and the irony was that illiterate white people could vote without worry.

On that glorious Sunday, hundreds of marchers headed toward Montgomery by way of the Edmund Pettus Bridge. To stop their effort, Governor, George Wallace allowed Alabama State Troopers to stand in their way and order them to turn around. Jim Clark, known to my family as Cotton, was a good friend of Pop's. He was also the sheriff responsible for so many repulsive and violent attacks on African American people. If marchers refused to turn around, his troopers were allowed to use nightsticks, tear gas, and bullwhips or, if they were mounted troops, their horses, to end the march.

Being a true Southern family normally means that decorum and presentation to the community is prized above all else. The appearance of being normal is of the utmost importance, regardless of how ridiculous the lie is to cover up the truth. If a family member is an alcoholic, it is not uncommon to hear they are "suffering from seizures" as the reason for their erratic behavior. I once went to a social function where a lady refused to wear her glasses because she didn't want anyone to know she required vision correction. She spent the entire time mistaking people and talking to random objects instead of putting on her glasses and embracing getting older. My family was no different.

My mother's parents met for the first time when Mema was only thirteen years old and Pop was twenty-six. Only five-feet tall with auburn hair, she had porcelain skin and clear blue eyes. Her dream was to be a Rockette at Radio City Music Hall, but instead she became a wife and homemaker.

She was a nurturer, but she could also be a determined and unapproachable adversary. A typical Southern housewife of her times, she could cook anything, and her meals were always absolutely delicious.

At six-feet four-inches, Pop was strong, burly, and aggressive, using his size and temper to get what he wanted. He was a significant member of the community and had a hand in everything involving local politics.

In my eyes, he was the walking devil with brown hair, blue eyes, and a nose so large and red that it looked more like a tumor than a nose. He always smelled like the electric shave lotion he used with his electric razor. Every time I would smell that aftershave it was like someone had opened up a bottle of fermenting orange juice.

Pop was one of twelve children, and not much is known in our family about his childhood, other than the fact that his family owned a lumber business. Growing up, he and his brothers would work out in the forest cutting trees and using Clydesdale Horses to bring the cut trees back to the logging facilities. I was told that his mother was insensitive and one of the meanest people many had ever met, which made me believe she was a big contributor as to why Pop is the way he is. Many times during one of his numerous sexual attacks on me, he would tell me to relax because he and his brother used to do this all the time.

Despite my sympathy and empathy for all those who endured sexual abuse, in my ruminations of his past I have come to realize that he remains without excuse for his behavior. The repeated and determined attempts to hide his actions indicate an understanding that they are wrong.

My mom has two older brothers. As the only girl, she was pampered and spoiled. Blonde and beautiful, she was paraded through all the right social circles and grew up to be one of the most popular girls in town. To this day, she is treated like "the baby," which is perhaps why she does not face adversity well or make sound adult decisions.

Dad's parents were wonderful and a bit unusual. Though my grandfather, whom we called Papaw, was eighteen years older than my grandmother, whom we called Momma O, they were soul mates from the time they met. A Native American princess, Momma O, had beautiful black hair, blue eyes, a flawless olive complexion and perfectly manicured finger nails, even up to her death.

My parents had bought a small house near their own for my Papaw and Momma O. A few months before passing away, I found some boxes filled with photographs at Papaw's house. I spent an entire day sitting in a porch swing going through the pictures of my grandparents, learning things about their lives I had never known before.

This is when I discovered that his marriage to Momma O was a second marriage for Papaw. His first wife had, unfortunately, died from an opium overdose. He was devoutly religious and very embarrassed by his first wife's death. We didn't even learn of the first marriage and her death until we found a box of old papers after he died.

Papaw was extremely intelligent and worked hard all his life. After his death, it was revealed that he had received a number of awards for coming up with formulas for the Pepsi Company. He came up with the formula for Old Dutch Chocolate Drink which he named after his company Old Dutch Bottling Company.

He kept all this to himself, never telling the family about his accomplishments. He was also a generous and caring man, and was the only white man who volunteered at a shelter for battered women.

Momma O was very different. It wasn't unusual to find her getting up at noon after drinking most of the night with her colleagues. She was the opposite of everything Papaw represented. Tall and beautiful, she smoked, drank, and reigned over a rough crowd of what could only be called thugs. She flaunted her money, thinking nothing of spending thousands of dollars on clothes and furniture in a single shopping spree.

She owned a restaurant that we loved to go to when we were children. She always made us delicious milkshakes. It was a classic American diner. It had chrome barstools with black seats that lined the counter area where we would always sit. She would see us coming and start the blenders and slide the glasses across the counter for us to stop them.

She also had a dark side. She got started in the loan-shark business because she did the payroll for Papaw's bottling company giving loans to the employees who couldn't make it from one paycheck to the next. These were paid back with interest or else she would get her guys to go to their house, bust open the door and take things to sell to pay her back.

She, of course, developed a reputation as someone good to do business with, and her reputation grew. She was well known in Selma as someone who would loan anyone money, but paying her back was a must. She had a few people who "worked with her" and helped enforce deadlines when loans needed to be paid back. Many times when I spent the night, I noticed that she always felt safer if I slept in the same room as she. At the foot of her bed was a big black purse, containing about ten thousand dollars and a gun. She was a colorful character; so much fun, and so fun loving to me.

Papaw, however, was a conservative Baptist deacon, a pillar in the community because of his volunteerism and deep-rooted civic involvement. Never before had a couple so epitomized the adage of opposites attracting. He and Momma O had two sons, my father and his brother, and a daughter that family legend says was found at a bus station by Papaw. My true suspicions are that she was from his first marriage, yet another example of the image-is-everything societal norm of the South.

Momma O's involvement in her loan shark business ended abruptly when she was in a near-fatal car accident. Coming home from an evening collection run, the car she was riding in swerved and flipped over several times. Since she was not wearing a seatbelt, she was thrown around inside the car before being thrown into the back seat.

She broke numerous bones and was treated with heavy-duty pain killers and prednisone, which made her bones brittle and caused her to developed rheumatoid arthritis and osteoporosis. She suffered from chronic pain for the rest of her days, but she lived into her eighties.

All of these things happened before my time. I was born in 1968, and because of the civil rights movement and the need for equality; Martin Luther King Jr. was my hero. I studied about him in school, and was simply amazed at his contributions to society, his efforts to make this world an equal and better place to live by overcoming hatred and bigotry. Today, I feel my passion for equality not only comes from great leaders like Martin Luther King Jr., but also from one of the most important people in my life, Nelly.

Nelly was Mema and Pop's maid, but to me she was more of a savior because of her tireless efforts to protect me. She invoked the same feelings of peace in me that most people would get from being curled up on a couch in front of a fire sipping hot cocoa. Like most domestic workers, she was aware of everything that was going on in their house. She was amazing to me and always tried to keep me occupied when Pop was around. She included me in almost all that she did just to keep me focused on other things and keep me at a distance from him.

I positively hated going to my grandparents' house except when I knew Nelly was there. She was my confidante, best friend, and the most amazing mentor I've ever had in my life. She taught me about individuality, how to stand up for myself, how to respect myself, and most importantly how to survive and still value myself in the end.

When I walked in the door of their home, Nelly was usually cleaning, doing laundry or folding clothes. She taught me how to sort clothes, making sure I put the right color combination into the right group. She also shared so many of her other talents to help me become an independent young man.

Nelly was about five feet tall, with smooth dark skin, high cheek bones, and a very serene demeanor. She was beautiful and perfect to me but no one else in my family could see past her ethnicity.

She reminded me of a tiny young Maya Angelou because of the peace and security that she exuded. She didn't have a lot of formal education, but when it came to knowing how to survive the rough spots in life, she was a scholar. My family viewed her as someone in the background, but she was very much in the lime light for me. She knew my family's secrets and never said a word to anyone. I believe this was because my family held her hostage financially. She had very little of her own and desperately needed the job she had with my family.

There were those in my family who said she was an alcoholic, but I would always yell back at them, saying, "No, she isn't."

Then Pop would smugly ask, sounding like the cartoon character Foghorn Leghorn, "Well, why do you think I have to drop her off at the liquor store all the time."

What everyone didn't know was Nelly and I talked about everything. She loved me and was the only person connected to my family who tried to protect me. I decided to ask her about being a "drunk," which was what my family called her among other things, and why she always asked Pop to drop her off at the liquor store.

She simply smiled, as she always did, and said, "Child, that's the only place that I can get him to drop me off so I can cash my check. I don't drink the devil's juice, but if that is what they want to believe, then that is just fine with me. I know who I am and I only have to answer to one person in this world, and that is me." *This is why I love her. She doesn't care what people think or say about her and I want to be that way too.*

Her simple eloquence showed me that it really doesn't matter what other people think of you as long as you think highly of yourself.

Sometimes I had to go to my grandparents' house after school because my mom had to work late or my dad had forgotten to pick us up. Nelly always volunteered to work late these evenings, hoping Mom would arrive before she had to leave. She did this because she knew what happened to me after Pop came home.

Pop often asked me if I'd like to ride along when he took Nelly home, and she usually tried to convince me to stay behind. I felt she knew the things he would force me to do after we dropped her off on the drive back to his house.

With the great racial divide so apparent in my grandparents' household, I can only imagine how difficult it must have been to be African American and work for such racist, angry people. Always true to her word, Nelly loved me unconditionally and never once made me feel any other way than perfect and protected.

As our relationship grew, she became aware of the pattern of abuse, and it became obvious to me that she wanted to do something to help. One afternoon, I had to use the bathroom, and Nelly was cleaning the one that I normally used. She told me to go to my grandparents' room and use the one in there.

It quickly became obvious to her that I was terrified to go into their room even though Pop wasn't due home from work for hours. I ran down into the den to make sure Mema was home because Pop was less likely to do something when she was there. As I ran through the kitchen I could hear my bare feet slap against the grey stone mosaic floor and down the steps into the den. I was relieved to see her sitting on the couch.

She looked at me and said, "What do you need?"

I told her that I was just checking to make sure someone was home, and I turned around and darted back upstairs. At this point my bladder felt like it was going to explode. I ran back through the kitchen, smiled and looked at Nelly and said, "I think the coast is clear, and I will be right back." She winked saying she would keep a look out for me.

I walked through the doorway of their room and past the foot of their bed, avoiding it like I would a land mine, rounded their dresser, and then walked into their bathroom. I was doing my potty dance as I shut the door and as soon as I lifted the lid—relief.

I didn't get to enjoy my relief long. It was interrupted by Pop's voice. I panicked. *What is he doing home already? It isn't even four o'clock!*

I tried to stop and I couldn't, so I tried to rush as quickly as I could, but it wasn't coming out fast enough. My heart was pounding and my panic grew. I heard Nelly in the hallway talking to him. It sounded like she was just talking about anything she could think of, her words just random.

He strode right past her as if he were in a hurry and came straight into his bedroom. I had closed the bathroom door, so I thought if I remained quiet, he wouldn't hear me. I pictured myself sneaking out as soon as he turned his back.

I tried to be as quiet as possible as I finished using the bathroom. I didn't want to flush the toilet because I didn't want to make any noise. I quietly put down the toilet lid and tiptoed to the wall of the bathroom. I placed my back against the wall beside the door which was slightly ajar. This gave me some perspective. I could look through the mirror on the opposite wall and see the movement taking place in their bedroom without being seen.

My eyes were glued to the mirror, but in my peripheral vision, I realized the bathroom window was open. I couldn't believe my luck! If I could find a way to open the screen without being heard, I might be able to climb out undetected. I looked at the mirror and didn't see anything going on nearby, so I walked slowly towards it.

Meanwhile, Nelly was doing everything that she could to distract him. I hoped he was in his bedroom changing clothes or doing something that would take him a few minutes. I slowly approached the window, and I realized that the opening would be very tricky to get out of.

This window was not a traditional bathroom window. It opened vertically, sliding from left to right. Directly below it was an empty towel bar. Slowly, I reached up to quietly unlatch the screen. Accidentally, I hit the towel bar and it made a loud clanking noise. I stopped . . . fear paralyzed me. I knew he had heard the noise because there was a pause in his conversation.

As I held my breath, I overheard Nelly telling Mema that Pop needed her in the bedroom. I finally exhaled and thought she was the smartest person in the world at that moment.

Mema came into the room and during their conversation I tried to move as quickly as I could to get the screen opened. I cautiously moved to avoid the towel bar and began struggling with the screen. I couldn't figure out how to open it and I didn't want to push it through because I was afraid it would make too much noise. I felt my way around and finally remembered that there was a safety latch. I grabbed the safety latch and pulled on it and the window screen slid open. I was so excited I put my foot on the wall and grabbed the edge of the window and began to pull myself up, trying to avoid the loud bar. I placed one foot on the ledge and as I went to pull my other foot up beside me, Pop opened the bathroom door.

He wore only his boxers, and he gave me a puzzled look as he said, "What in the world are you doing?"

I guess that during all of my planning I didn't hear Mema leave the room or hear him walking into the bathroom. I looked at him and said the first things that popped into my head, "Oh, I heard you in your room, and I didn't want to bother you, so I decided to just climb out the window."

He grabbed my arm like a bear trap and said, "Get back in here."

He gave me a hard jerk, and I landed against him instead of on the floor. Big eyed and feeling like I had just been placed in a cage for a fight against someone double my size, I started to pull away, thinking I could just pretend I appreciated his help and get away.

He leaned over, pressing his body weight against me, pinning me to the wall as he shut the screen and the window. The same towel bar that I tried so hard to avoid was now being forced into my back. It felt as if my spinal cord was going to be snapped in half from the pressure. Almost in one movement he yanked the shade down, and reached around to lock the bathroom door.

I could feel the slight reprieve of his body pressure and squirmed my way out from his clench. I darted and grabbed for the door knob, as I did, I kicked the door and it flung open. He pushed me down on the carpet in the bedroom and grabbed me by the back of the head while pulling his boxer shorts down.

He grabbed my face and said, "I came home early to get me some of this."

With that, he shoved his penis in my face. I started crying and begged him to *please* stop. *I should just bite his dick off,* I thought to myself but afraid he would kill me if I refrained.

He gave me a cold look and said, "But I thought you liked me to do this."

"Why would you think that?" I asked through my tears.

Suddenly the door opened and Nelly stepped inside like she didn't know he was in the room. I tried to lunge toward her but his grip was so tight on my neck it felt like a brace and I couldn't even move my head. My eyes were turned as far to the corner as I could get them and I made contact with her and then I felt a tear roll down my cheek. He looked at her and said, "You stupid nigger, shut the damn door."

Of course she had no choice. She did what he said, and he finished with me. I was sobbing and feeling numb at the same time. He was such a monster. After he was done, he got dressed, and I just sat in the same spot, starring at the floor in disbelief.

He walked out and went down into the den and kissed Mema as if it was just another day in his life.

Nelly came running into the room, and I collapsed into her arms, crying and crying, asking her why he did these horrible things to me. She looked at me and said, "Because he knows he can, that's why. Now, you need to pull yo'self together, and meet me outside in the shed."

The shed was on the corner of my grandparent's property in the back yard. It was built out of plywood and had the distinct odor of oil and gasoline. Pop stored all of his lawn equipment, motorcycles and yard tools there. It was the only place Nelly and I felt safe to talk when he was home. It was shadowed by a huge pecan tree, so it was never hot inside.

I got up, straightened my clothes, and walked through the house and outside to the shed. Even at the age of nine, I knew we had to be discreet in how and where we spoke to each other because Pop had no appreciation for her as a person because of her race. Every time she and I spoke we ran the risk of getting pummeled by him. My grandparents of course felt that she needed to only focus on work, and not interacting with me. Naturally, Nelly never once considered that a big concern for herself. All she cared was that I was as all right as the situation would allow.

She finished cleaning the bathroom and walked outside to throw out the dirty water she had been using to mop the floor. She quickly walked behind the shed, with one look over her shoulder, stepped through the door.

She quietly shut the door, turned around with tears in her eyes and said, "Please don't think you did anything to deserve this, because you didn't. That man is just the devil himself, and I will do everything I can to protect you," she said, her voice low but determined.

I just enjoyed feeling her arms around me. She always smelled like Cocoa Butter and the scent had become so embracing. I knew she would protect me as best she could. When she spoke again, she said, "I will have a talk with your grandmother. I know she will do something about it, I just know she will."

I believed her because I didn't have any other options.

The following week, I overheard Nelly confronting Mema regarding her concerns about Pop's actions. She approached it in a very indirect way, saying, "Mrs. Jowers, if someone was hurting one of yo' grandchilen', wouldn't you want to know about it?"

"Of course I would," Mema responded immediately.

"What if it was someone that you knew?" Nelly asked quietly.

"I cannot imagine anyone we know who would hurt any of my grandkids," she said, defensively.

"What if I told you I seen it with my own two eyes?"

"Nelly, what do you know, and why haven't you said anything before now?"

"Because I don't want to lose my job," Nelly said flatly.

"If someone is hurting my grandchildren, then you must tell me who it is. You are my eyes, and I cannot think of anyone that has come around here who would hurt them."

"It is someone who is not a visitor; it is someone who lives here." It was as if she were talking to the floor. She refused to lift her head and make eye contact and both of her hands were behind her back. I could hear the fear in her voice.

"The only people who live here are Mr. Jowers and myself," she said dismissively.

"Yes, ma'am." Her eyes lifted slowly from the floor to support the fact that she had just guessed the answer correctly.

Looking confused she questioned. "So, are you saying that Mr. Jowers has hurt the children?"

"Yes, ma'am." Her eyes immediately went directly back to the floor and her shoulders hunched over slightly. She was feeling conquered with what she was hoping to accomplish.

"How?" Her brows were furrowed and her tone was curt.

I could hear the fear in her voice and I was so frightened for her and so very thankful at the same time.

"Mrs. Jowers, I walked into yo' bedroom to put up the clothes I had folded, and when I opened the door, he had Geebo down on the floor, holding his head and forcing his thing into the child's mouth," Nelly said. "When I looked at him, he told me to get out of the room. When I looked at Geebo, he had tears running down his little face and his blue eyes were the size of saucers. I am so sorry that I waited this long to tell you, but I was afraid of what Mr. Jowers may do or say."

Geebo was the nickname given to me by my sister. To this day, I can't stand being called that because of all these types of memories.

With her hands on her hips and an attitude that was more vicious than I had ever heard before she said, "You stupid drunk nigger, how could you say something like that against my husband?"

"But Mrs. Jowers…" Nelly's eyes quickly rose from the floor and her hands moved from behind her back ready to block any punch that may come her way.

Mema quickly spun around and venomously said "Nelly, I think it would be best if you collect your things, and I will have Mr. Jowers take you home,"

"But Mrs. Jowers," Nelly pleaded, "what he has done is not right." She reached out towards Mema to put her hands on her arm to get her to understand. She quickly pulled her arm away and raised it into the air to strike her. Nelly cowed down fearing the worst and Mema lowered her hand and placed them conservatively in front of her.

Without emotion she proceeded. "He has not done anything, and if you value your job and what you are paid, you will not breathe a word of this. Honestly, after all that we have done for you, why would you want to say such terrible things?" Mema's voice was haughty now.

Nelly slowly turned and walked into the living room and grabbed the bag she always brought with her every morning. I walked up to her as she started collecting her things, still crying. She knelt down and put her hands on my face and said, "I am so sorry, I tried to let her know what I know, but she don't believe me and I'm afraid they never will."

I looked at her and said, "Please don't cry. I don't want you not to be here anymore. I want you to stay."

"I will do my best to protect you while I am here but that is all I will be able to do," Nelly said as she finished packing her bag.

She was my guardian angel and the only person who loved me enough to care about confronting them. To think she was considered less than a second class citizen to them but to me she was as first class as a person could get.

The next day I came running home after school because I knew Nelly would be there and I could tell her all about my day and give her the craft I made for her in class. When I got close to the front door, I could smell the wonderful aromas of her food and the scent of bleach from the washing machine, so I knew she was working.

Knowing Pop would not be home and we could talk anywhere, I burst through the front door and set out to find her. I went into the family room, then to the kitchen, then to the living room, and I couldn't find her. I saw Mema sitting at the kitchen table, and I asked her if she had seen Nelly.

She replied sternly, "She is in the bathroom, and as soon as she takes care of her personal business, she needs to get to work, so don't bother her today."

I went running to the bathroom. As I hurried down the hallway, I heard Nelly moan, and I wondered what she was doing. The bathroom door was slightly ajar and as I peeked through the opening I could see that she was throwing up blood! I went running back to the kitchen, screaming at Mema, "Nelly is dying. She is on the bathroom floor, and she is throwing up blood!"

Mema continued to sit at the table with a blank look on her face. I burst into tears and began screaming at her, "Did you hear me? I think she is dying."

She told me to stay away from Nelly because she was just a drunk and that there was nothing we could do.

I couldn't believe the indifference she was displaying. I was afraid that I had caused this to her.

I ran into the bathroom and grabbed Nelly's hand. She looked at me and told me she would be fine, not to worry about her. I told her that I had to worry about her because she was the only friend I had.

Mema then came in and pushed me aside, telling Nelly to get up off of the floor. I looked at Mema and told her I was going to call an ambulance. She grabbed me by the arm like the thorns on a rose bush with her finger nails almost piercing the skin on my forearm and told me not to worry about it, because she called Pop. He was on his way home to take Nelly to the hospital.

I told Nelly not to worry that Pop was on his way and that I would go with her to the hospital. I ran from the bathroom to the front door to see if he was home yet. Every time I went back into the bathroom, I could tell Nelly was getting weaker and weaker. When I came back the last time, she had fallen over and could no longer sit up. Realizing that she was helpless, she the only person that would protect me, it was now my turn to protect her.

It was at least thirty minutes before Pop finally got home and I didn't understand why. Even I knew you could drive from one end of Selma to the other within ten minutes. As he opened the door, I ran up to him and started pulling on his hand.

"Please hurry up. I don't think she is doing very well."

He looked at me with coldness in his eyes and said, "Where is Mema?"

"I don't know. I have been with Nelly. Please, please help me get her into the car," I said, feeling my fear growing.

While I was trying to get Nelly out of the bathroom, I was wondering where Pop had gone because I was so sure he knew how serious her condition was. He went to find Mema, who was downstairs watching TV. It was her habit to sit in front of the television for hours just listening pretending she could see.

I went back into the bathroom and tried with all of my strength to pull Nelly down the hallway. She weighed about ninety pounds, but I was only about seventy pounds myself. Pop finally came back and pushed me out of the way. He picked Nelly up and carried her to the car. As he lifted her up, her head fell back. She was completely lifeless and her limbs just dangled. I thought she was dead.

He got her into the car and as I crawled into the backseat, he glared at me and in a low intense, deep voice sneered, "get out of the car." Confused why he was telling me this I didn't flinch. I looked at him and said, "I have to go with her because I promised her I would." Unwavering with his choice he retorted back, "You need to take care of Mema while I drive her to the hospital." Because Nelly was so sick, I didn't want to waste any time arguing.

I ran inside to the family room where she still sat watching television. "How can you be so calm?" I asked

She said, "I think she must have been bitten by a spider or something."

"What kind of spider? I thought you said she was sick because she was drunk." Nothing was making sense now. I waited and finally said, "Do you know what happened to her?"

"Stop asking so many questions," was all she said.

I tried to be quiet, but it was clear to me that she knew more about what was going on than I did. Without thinking I said, "Do you think she will be all right?"

She just sat there and completely ignored me, continuing to listen to her program.

A short while later, Pop pulled into the driveway, and I could see Nelly was not in the car. I burst out the front door like a bullet from a fired gun, asking questions as I went.

"How is she? What happened? Where is she? Did she die?"

He walked past me muttering, "Don't worry. I'm sure she'll be fine."

"You mean you don't know what happened to her," I said with astonishment.

"I said she will be fine, so leave me alone."

As he walked passed me I just stood there watching the evening sun start to set trying to imagine what was going through her mind and how scared she was. I wanted to be with her so badly, but I knew that even if I went up to the hospital, they wouldn't let me see her. I didn't even know her last name. I knew so much about her, but I didn't know this one crucial detail.

I guess it was an hour or so after Pop arrived back at the house that the phone rang. My Aunt Dolly called, and I heard her say, "Grace, [Mema's real name] Nelly is at the hospital. Did you know?"

Mema took the phone into the kitchen, her voice sounding weak and timid. "Yes, we knew she was there. Bernard is the one who took her to the hospital."

She went on to tell my aunt that she had been doing nothing but taking care of Nelly all afternoon because of a terrible mistake. Nelly had been cleaning in the bathroom and somehow had ingested some of the chemicals she mixed.

I had no idea what "ingested" meant, but I could only imagine. Mema continued to talk, saying how terrible it was and adding, "I helped her in the bathroom the entire day, and Bernard got home early so he could rush her to the hospital. You have no idea what I have been through this afternoon. And poor Geebo, he had to witness the entire thing."

I listened to her affected southern drawl and wondered if I had just imagined everything that had happened since I came home. What did she mean by mixing chemicals? I thought Nelly was either drunk or got bit by a spider? I didn't witness anything. All I felt was confused and frustrated. And everything was becoming more and more confusing. All I wanted to do was go to the hospital and make sure Nelly was all right.

Three weeks later Nelly returned to my grandparents' house, and I couldn't wait to see her. Like always when she was there, I could smell the aroma of her delicious cooking and the hint of bleach from her doing the laundry. This time I cautiously opened the door and gingerly walked across the family room, then into the kitchen, where she was at the sink washing dishes.

I went running up to her and threw my arms around her waist. I was so happy to see her, and as I hugged her, she looked over her shoulder to see if

Mema could hear us. She bent on one knee, looked into my face and said, "I really need to do my work today so I will have to talk to you later on. I missed a lot of time away, and I have a lot of cleaning to do."

I looked in her eyes and I could see the fear. It was the same fear I would see in my face when I looked in the mirror after I was abused. It closely resembled a person who had been put on the frontline of a war without a gun. I had felt that same confusion in the horrifying moments with Pop when I would be trying to figure out how I was going to survive. I completely understood what she was talking about. From that day, I rarely had the opportunity to spend a lot of time with Nelly because she was so frightened of what my grandparents might do to her.

One day while she was outside hanging out clothes on the clothesline, I sneaked around and hid behind a sheet so I could talk to her. I asked her about that awful day and if she had been bitten by a spider. She said no, so I asked her if she were so drunk she started throwing up, and she gave me one of her famous looks that told me I was being ridiculous.

She looked at me and said, "Where in the world did you get these silly ideas from?"

I told her it was what Mema had told me. Her face went as hard as stone, but she said nothing. Finally I asked her what happened. She looked at me and said she couldn't really talk about it, that maybe one day I would understand. I took her words at face value because I knew she would never lie to me, and she also knew what was best. I then looked at her and said "I have one very important question for you, what is your last name?" She relaxed her face and smiled cheek to cheek and said "Johnson."

As time passed, it became more and more difficult for us to spend time together because of her fear of my grandparents. I always found creative ways to involve myself with her work so she was forced to speak with me. When we were able to be together, we would just laugh and talk for hours, and it would make all of my pain go away, as if life were perfect.

Mema always found us. She would look at me and say, "Don't bother her while she is working. We don't pay her to talk."

It never stopped me because I just ignored her just as she did Nelly that day and continued my conversation, pretending I didn't hear her.

Nelly continued to work for my grandparents throughout my adolescence, though my contact with her was very limited. After my mother and I moved away from Selma, I was not allowed to talk to her again. I still miss her and long for our talks together. She was a beautiful person in every possible way, and I am who I am today because of what she instilled in me.

CHAPTER 3

THE MORE THEY STAY THE SAME

There were times in my life when I thought things would change for me and the abuse would end. The summer after my fourth grade in school, Dad got a promotion and we moved to Mobile. At last, I was getting away from Selma, the hatred and abuse from Pop, which was astoundingly exciting. The one thing that I would also be getting away from is the only person who had shown me what unconditional love was all about – Nelly. It was a double-edged sword. She was my safety net and the only security I had ever known, but she would not be able to go with us. I was nervous because of the change, and excited at the opportunity to start a new life where no one knew us.

This move was proving to be one of the best things that had ever happened to me. I began making new friends and really enjoying school for the first time. I joined the key club, the football team, and even volunteered as a safety crossing guard. I thought it was amazing, even though everyone else thought I was a dork.

The only members of my family in Mobile were my mom, Dad, and my sister Evelyn, so it was wonderful! What I didn't know was my parents were struggling to keep their marriage together. They kept it hidden well, and kept their children out of their arguments. Occasionally, I heard Mom crying through their bedroom door, but overall, it wasn't distressing.

Dad traveled a lot, so the thought of him being gone long-term wasn't too bothersome.

Our subdivision was new and as more homes were built, I made more friends. My parents started doing more "couples" things to try and save their marriage, and my sister and I were home alone a lot. It was OK, because I could visit my science teacher, who lived next door, and just down the street were my best friends, Keith and Marissa. I was ten years old and in fourth grade, finally experiencing a sense of individuality and independence.

One day as I walked down to Keith's house I remember purposefully taking in a deep breath and smelling the fresh cut grass and looking around at all of the beautifully built homes. *This is perfect, I have friends who really seem to accept me and I don't have to worry about anything but school. I love it here!*

We went to a neighborhood school, and we all walked to school as a group every morning. My teachers were interesting and, since no one knew my family, I was free to be me without worry of being judged or of being bothered by Pop.

My sister made a lot of friends too, and she'd have slumber parties with a lot of the neighborhood kids that were her age. We were both enjoying ourselves and made great grades. It felt like for the first time ever we were truly happy and healthy, because we didn't have my grandfather nearby to interfere with our family.

In an effort to gain acceptance from my dad, I tried out for basketball and made the first two cuts. I came running home and exploded through the front door *"Dad, I know you are going to love this, I made the second cut,"* as I jumped up and hit my fingers on the top of the door frame.

He turned around and had the proudest smile on his face. *Our final practice is tomorrow and I just know I am going to make it.* The next day we played our last scrimmage game and had the coaches pick their draft choices. We were told we would find out the results by the end of the day, and I waited with anticipation, running to the gym after my last class of the day. As I ran into the gym that smelled like sweaty socks, I pushed my way through all of the other kids who were also anxiously awaiting their results.

You could hear the excitement from some and the disappointment from the others. I finally got to the front of the line. *I know he is going to be so proud of me, I just know I made the team,* I chanted to myself. As I scanned the list I didn't see my name and realized I didn't make the team. With both disbelief and disappointment, I was scared to go home to tell him. I just knew he would once again think that I was not good enough. I was right. His lack of acceptance hurt but it didn't discourage me. I thought it was great that I made the first two cuts. It would have been nice to hear that from Dad but his lack of acknowledgement fueled my drive to succeed even more.

I was gaining confidence by playing sports, sometimes succeeding and sometimes failing. It was a confidence I'd never had before. When football season rolled around, I decided to see what I could do with that.

I tried out for the football team, hoping to both redeem myself with Dad and reclaim some self respect with my classmates. I made the first two cuts without any problems and then the third time I received a call at home telling me that I had made the team. *Finally, I have a chance to prove to him that I am as good as all of the other kids.*

I played center and right guard. I was on top of the world. I was popular, playing sports, and making more great friends. Dad offered to coach my football team. I was hesitant at first, *does he want to coach me because he thinks I can't do a good job without him, or is it because he also wants us to have a better relationship?*

I know he wanted only the best for me, but once he started coaching me, he became a rigid personal trainer. He explained that my diet needed to change. I had no idea what he meant but once I got home my first meal after making the team consisted of a hamburger patty and brown rice and that was about it. He measured my meat portions and refused to allow me anything more even if I was starving.

Every night after dinner he insisted we run and burn off the calories I'd just eaten! He wanted to keep my weight at ninety pounds for game weigh-in days because of strict size regulations for the ages of the kids we played against. I had become a very good player and he didn't want to run the risk of me not being able to play because of a weight restriction. I didn't mind all of Dad's new rules because I was really enjoying the attention and thought it would be good for me anyway.

I was now eleven years old, the tallest kid in my class, and had a never-ending appetite. I remember checking out other people's lunch trays to see if there were any pieces of uneaten food left because I was constantly starving. By the end of the first season, I was experiencing severe stomach pains and even went through periods where I could barely get out of bed. Mom would come in, like she did every morning to wake me, and flip on my bedroom light, *please let this be a terrible nightmare,* but instead it was time to get ready for school.

Dad always said I was faking the pain, stating that it was all in my head. He continuously accused me of losing interest in the game.

I worked hard to push myself and please him. At the end of the season, picture day arrived, and I got dressed in my uniform. The last thing I wanted to do that day was smile for a camera. I was doubled over with a pain that had shifted from hunger to the most intense stabbing feeling. Standing up straight was a near impossibility. When I would finally reach the complete erect position, I would just fold again due to the powerful sting that I felt in my side.

Dad was so proud of me, and I wanted to make sure I continued to make him happy, so I didn't mention a word of how I was feeling to him. I didn't want to hear again that I was faking it, or how I was doing this as a ploy to avoid having my picture taken.

The entire drive all I could do was think about the stabbing pain in my side. *If I can just make it there and try and smile for the picture this will all be over.* After Dad shifted the car into park I opened the car door and grabbed my football from the back seat. I became really dizzy and started seeing black dots as I fell to one knee, *I am okay,* I said to myself acting as if I had slipped on something.

We made it across the field and I looked at the camera person, "Are you okay," the camera guy asked.

"Yes I am fine, where do I need to go?"

I was not really interested in doing anything but getting this day over with. I wanted to get back home to take off all of this ridiculously hot gear. I was trying not to be too dismissive but I really didn't care.

"Walk over there by the football helmet and just hold the football like you are running for a touchdown"

I looked up and saw the red helmet he had mentioned and started walking. I got positioned behind it and with a "one, two, three smile" the camera snapped.

My smile was more of a strain from the pain, but regardless I think we are done.

"Do I need to do anything else or are you done?"

"Great job, see you next year," He said as he started loading his film for the next guy behind me.

Only if I live to next year, I thought.

Once we got back home I peeled off the sweaty football uniform and fell into bed. Mom came in to check on me, yet I could not come out of the fetal position.

"Mom, I think I am dying," I whispered, saying it as if I had marbles in my mouth.

She had a concerned look on her face and she gently placed her hand on my forehead. Alarmed that I felt so warm, she started to help me up so I could get dressed. "You are burning up with a fever."

I tried to focus on her face but didn't have the energy and just fell onto her shoulder. She propped me up against the wall and put a pair of shorts on me that were at the foot of my bed. I had just taken them off because I was so hot. Slowly she pulled my body weight onto the floor and leaned me up against her.

She was screaming for Dad to come and help her but he was no where around. He had dropped me off and left without letting anyone know.

"I am going to take you to the emergency room." She said as her eyes changed from concern to fear.

We walked down the hallway, into the kitchen where Mom grabbed her car keys. We walked out of the back door of the house and sped off to the Mobile Infirmary. She was not a doctor by any stretch of the imagination, but felt certain it was an appendicitis attack. Once we arrived into the parking lot she pulled the car into the first available spot she could see. She snatched her purse from beside her and came running around to my door to help me out.

As the door handle clicked, I could feel the cool air from outside of the car slowly blow across my face. She pulled me carefully to my feet, being sympathetic knowing how difficult it was for me to stand straight. "Remember how you walked up against me at home, well, do that again." I looked at her and just collapsed up against her as she slowly walked me through the automatic sliding doors. I heard the swoosh sound of the doors open and could feel the rush of the frigid air against my body which caused me to convulse with chills. "Hang in there we are almost where we need to be," She said encouragingly. We walked up to a desk where a lady sat and Mom began giving her all of our insurance information.

The emergency room nurse took one look at me and sent us straight back to see the doctor. Within an hour they had admitted me. The doctors were concerned because the pain in my abdominal area was so intense at times I almost would become unconscious. The diagnosis was a stomach ulcer, and the doctor was concerned. It was the first time they had seen an ulcer in someone so young.

How can I break this news to Dad and still have him like me? I was frightened that things would never be the same and they indeed were not.

He came to the hospital to see me and could barely look me in the face. When he finally did, I could see that there was complete disappointment and disgust in his eyes. I knew I had let him down as a son and as a football player. Needless to say, I never put myself in a situation where Dad could be my coach again.

Aside from the occasional hospital visits, our first year in Mobile was great. We loved our neighborhood, and most of the kids were on the same sports teams and involved in the same after-school activities. I was very happy, but I wasn't so sure about Evelyn.

Growing up, she was somewhat of a tomboy and a rebel. She always went against the grain of society by smoking, drinking and experimenting with drugs. I think it was because she was highly intelligent, more so than most of her peers and probably even some of her teachers. Her intelligence was only surpassed by her beauty. Her hair was long and the color of honey, eyes were like two blue marbles and her skin was of a rich olive complexion that was as close to perfect as anything I had ever seen.

As far back as I can remember, she was getting into trouble. One night while Dad was working late, Mom received a phone call from the local grocery store manager. He had just caught Evelyn shoplifting beer. Mom was so embarrassed, because she was always doing stuff like this. True to form, Evelyn would make up elaborate lies to get out of it. She had an uncanny ability to convince others she was right. Though we didn't realize it at the time, it was a survival tool that would aid her in her future.

I loved her and, in her own way, she loved me too and was incredibly protective. She defended me when I was picked on at school, but, like most sisters, had no qualms about picking on me herself at home. Our relationship as siblings was always tumultuous and since we've become adults, it is still somewhat strained.

Teachers were at a loss about how to treat Evelyn or how to punish her. She was normally bored and paid little attention in class, yet always made straight A's. There were weekly visits to the principal's office, but little was done because she was an honor roll student and a star athlete on the girls' softball and basketball teams.

Evelyn was barely seventeen, drinking, doing drugs, and going out of town without telling my parents where she was going. One night she called home, and it was obvious she was extremely drunk. She told my dad she was in Texas with Desiree, her best friend at the time, and that she had been raped. All Dad did was ask if she had a way to get back home.

How could she do this to them after everything they have done for her and continue to do for her? I would constantly ask myself when my parents were trying to save my sister from another situation she had gotten herself into.

When she finally got home, she told me she and Desiree had been at a bar where the bartender had given them free drinks all evening. When Evelyn decided to go back to their room and go to bed, Desiree didn't want to leave so Evelyn left without her.

Evelyn got up from her bar stool and stumbled her way through the lobby over to the bank of elevators. She pressed the button and suddenly heard a door slam behind her. As she turned to see if someone was there she became distracted by the elevator arriving to take her back to her room. Once she stopped on her floor and exited the doors she started walking down the hallway with an exaggerated swagger. She noticed that someone was behind her. As she looked over her shoulder she realized it was the bartender from downstairs. She thought nothing about it at first because he'd been friendly with her and Desiree all evening. When she finally reached her room door she spun around and sultrily asked, "Are you following me?" He put his hands on each side of her head and brought his face closer to hers. She was thrilled with excitement and then everything abruptly changed. With her eyes still closed she could feel his fingers slowly gripping around her throat. He demanded that she open the door.

She did what he said and once they were inside the room, he threw her down on the floor and she could feel the fibers of the carpet scrape against her face. He leaned in and started tearing her clothes off. Evelyn said she was so drunk she couldn't fight him. Once he was done, she lay there on the floor, partially clothed and in disbelief, praying she would not get pregnant because he did not use a condom. That's how my sister lost her virginity, at the tender age of seventeen.

That summer we got new neighbors across the street. They were the talk of the neighborhood. They were the quintessential family. He was a cop, she was a beautiful, and they had twin girls and a younger son. The Television show *Magnum P.I.* was a big hit then because of the sex appeal of the leading star, Tom Selleck, and that was how everyone referred to him.

His name was Dirk and he was hairy with a full mustache and a muscular body. Most of all, he was a cop, which made all of the women swoon. His wife, Tiffany, was as good looking as he was. She seemed eccentric to me because she did things most people didn't. When she wanted to lose weight, instead of dieting, she had her mouth wired shut. She was an executive and definitely the breadwinner in the family. She was funny and beautiful and I liked her because she liked me just the way I was. She listened to me, showed interest in the things I liked, and was very forgiving anytime I made a mistake.

Her daughters, Joan and Jane, were younger than I but we quickly became inseparable. Tiffany didn't seem to mind. I was hungry for attention from an adult, and she gave it to me. I grew to love her as I would a parent.

About a year after they moved in, Dirk and Tiffany began having problems in their marriage. Dirk met a girl when he was in St. Thomas Islands and had an affair. He and Tiffany tried to work through this rough patch, but he seemed more interested in going back to St. Thomas to visit his new girlfriend.

Tiffany was a feisty person, and it really didn't take long for her to get frustrated. She packed up her kids and moved out. He was left living alone in their huge house. I saw Joan, Jane, and little Dirk Jr., the youngest, when they visited, but that was not very often. Because they were so close to us and my after school and weekend visits had become a regular habit, I missed them terribly.

One Saturday night Dirk asked Mom if I could baby sit little Dirk and the twins while he went out for the evening. She said sure, and I looked forward to a night with friends.

When I arrived, I found only little Dirk had come, and he was already in bed. Dirk gave me instructions, told me where he was going, and left phone numbers on the refrigerator in case I needed him. He ordered me pizza and left me some cash for the delivery guy. He looked at me, winked and said, "Don't worry; it's not coming out of your baby-sitting money."

I wasn't worried at all because I hadn't known I was being paid. I enjoyed being away from my house, especially since all I had to do was watch TV and check on little Dirk while he slept.

I got my pizza, watched television, and cleaned the kitchen. I pretended the house was mine, and I was the adult taking care of everything. My belly was full and I was starting to get sleepy, so I made one last lap through the house to check on the baby. Their house was laid out almost identical to ours, so I didn't even turn on any lights. I looked in on little Dirk and I was able to see that he was still sound asleep because of the glow of the night lights that really lit up the room. As I stood in the doorway and looked at his perfect face I thought *"what an incredibly lucky kid he is to have such great parents that protect him and love him so much. If there were a way to recapture my life at his age, I would do it in a second."*

With everything in order, I headed back to the living room couch to finish my evening watching HBO. I began watching a movie and within twenty minutes, I was sound asleep.

When Dirk drove up, he woke me out of a sound sleep. I was afraid someone was trying to break in to the house, and I got scared. I looked for a weapon, and then suddenly the door flung open and Dirk stumbled in.

He was drunk and falling all over the place, so I helped him back to his bedroom. As we walked down the hall he mumbled about all women being bitches and how he was better off without them. He said some other things, but they were slurred so badly they weren't comprehendible.

I opened his bedroom door, and he fell across the bed. I slid his legs around and pulled the blanket up over his body. I told him I was going home, and he looked at me and said with repulsive liquor on his breath, "You are a great kid. Thanks."

The next morning I went back over there because I was concerned that little Dirk would wake up and he would still be asleep. I didn't want the little guy to get hurt. As soon as I arrived, I saw the back door was still unlocked.

Wait a second, when I left last night I know for sure that I locked the door because I remembered I would need their key this morning to get back inside.

I walked into the house that looked exactly like I'd left it the night before except little Dirk's belongings were no longer beside the recliner. I hoped his mother had picked him up earlier.

I tip toed down the hallway trying not to wake anyone and, just as I had thought, little Dirk wasn't there, so I headed to his dad's bed room. He was groggy but awake and told me Tiffany had picked up little Dirk earlier that morning.

He looks like a fifty year old man and smells like a cigarette factory, I thought to myself. The reality was he had just turned thirty five, and the stench was from the smoke from the night before.

I asked him if he was all right and sat down on the edge of the bed while we spoke. He said he was fine but asked me to get him a glass of water, which I did, from the kitchen.

As I returned to his bed room I questioned myself on what to do. *Should I go and get my parents to take care of him just in case he is really sick, because I do not know anything about how to take care of someone who has a hangover?*

When I returned to his room, he was lying on his stomach. Because of my history with my grandfather, I became frightened.

Just don't be so paranoid, I said to myself as I walked in looking at him as if he were a corpse.

He asked me to put the glass of water on the nightstand. I did and began backing toward the door.

He was a cop and I know he would not do anything to me, as I continued my self talk to keep me from freaking out.

I said, "I'll see you later," as I backed away.

He gently grabbed my arm and said, "There's one more thing I need you to do for me."

My heart started to beat at a ridiculously rapid pace and I could feel my stomach start to knot up inside like I was going to throw up.

He handed me a bottle of lotion and asked me to rub it on his shoulders.

Well, surely he wouldn't do anything to me because at school they told us that if you ever have any problems to go to a police officer because they had to take an oath to protect and serve, I still continued with this mental banter.

He couldn't reach them himself, he said, the sun had made his skin dry.

That makes sense, I thought to myself because his wife is no longer in his life.

I was relieved because it looked like he didn't want to do anything sexual.

I began rubbing the lotion, which smelled like coconuts and reminded me of the wonderful times we had when we would go on vacations, on my palms and then put it on his shoulders.

"This smell reminds me of the time I went to Panama City with my family. We used a suntan lotion that was like this," I said to fill the silent air.

I thought it was a little weird, but I justified it in my head by thinking he did live alone and there was no one else to do it for him. When I touched his skin, he let out a soft moan like he was feeling relief from a wonderful massage.

He began talking quietly in his smoky sounding voice, "thank you for doing such a great job last night with little Dirk. He really seems to like you." This actually put me at ease. Pop had never talked to me, so it helped calm my fear. He continued talking about how much he missed his kids and asked me if I had ever been down to St. Thomas Islands with my family. Nothing he talked about made me feel threatened. I finished and patted him on the arm to let him know I was done.

Why was I so scared? I thought to myself, *He is a nice, well-liked guy and I should be more trusting.*

He asked in the same easy voice, "Do you mind rubbing it down my back for me? I can't reach there either."

My intuition kicked in big time, and my mouth got very dry. I began to worry.

Okay, maybe I don't need to be so trusting and I should just leave but I don't want him to think that I don't like him especially because of all of the hard times he has had lately I don't want him to feel uncomfortable.

So I said sure, and gave him the benefit of the doubt. As I started down his back, he pulled the covers down lower, and I saw he was completely nude.

He reached up and shut the door and said he needed me to put lotion on his front side.

I can't believe he wants me to do this, I thought he was a nice guy and a great father to little Dirk. I was wanting little Dirk's life last night and now he is no different than Pop!

I asked why because I felt pretty confident he could reach that part of his body. He said it was because he was a cop and he asked me to do it. My heart was pounding and my body began to shake uncontrollably from nervousness.

Fearing he would make up something and put me in jail if I didn't do what he said, I began rubbing lotion on his stomach. I began inching my hands towards his groin area rubbing lotion sparsely along the path I was creating.

As, I rubbed the lotion on him I could feel my body shift from trembling to calm. I started to shut down and I could feel myself separate from the experience as if I were an outsider looking in.

I turned my head away from him and focused my eyes on the wall. He grabbed my hand and lowered it to his penis, and I thought I was going to throw up. I kept my focus on the wall and then I felt his other hand grab the back of my head and he pushed me down onto his penis.

I thought to myself, *well, this is just some hell, my mouth is full of coconut lotion and I was trying to do the right thing by coming over to check on them.* I prayed the entire time, and when he was finished I ran into the bathroom and threw up. I looked into the mirror as I saw the anger on my face and said to my reflection, *why are you doing this to me God?* I couldn't believe what happened there, and I felt as if it were surreal. I did not realize at the time how statistically common it is for an abused person to be molested again.

He rolled over when I came out of the bathroom and said, "If you tell anyone about this, I will take you straight to jail, no questions asked." I looked at him as if to say, *I know the freaking drill here, so don't worry.*

I felt somewhat relieved that he wasn't a family member and didn't threaten to kill someone. I left and walked across the street to our house, ran inside, turned on the shower and just sat in the corner of the tub curled up in a ball, unable to cry.

Is everything I went through in Selma going to happen to me again here? Not if my life had to end today would I allow this to happen to me again. I never told anyone. However, after that, I became reclusive because I just didn't want to go outside any more, out of self-protection.

My parents bought "play clothes" just to encourage me to go outside, and I would go home and change into them and go out onto the porch corner so they would think I was playing. In reality, I was wondering if what happened with Dirk and Pop was what life is all about. Thanks, but I'd rather stay inside and play with my horse figurines and my hamster.

When I did go outside, all I would do is play with my dog Lucky. Lucky was given to me by Papaw two days after I was born. He had found her abandoned under a house in a very depressed side of town. The owners had basically thrown her away. She was just a puppy, and we named her Lucky because she was lucky that we found her and saved her life. But I felt I was the lucky one because of her. She followed me everywhere, and she was always so very happy to see me.

I use to pretend that if she was a person, she would have long black hair and blue eyes and make all of the other people at school jealous because of her loyalty to me.

Finally, *my* luck changed too. Dirk moved away, and all I could think was *thank God, I didn't have to worry about going to jail anymore.* I never saw Dirk or his family again.

My parents continued to have difficulty with their marriage, and decided that they needed to be alone in order to repair things. They asked my sister and me if we would like to spend the summer with Mema and Pop.

My spirit sank; *I wish they understood how punishing those words sounded to me. I would do **anything** not to have to go back there, just please not there!*

I knew I couldn't stand an entire summer of abuse and mind games from my grandfather. I told my parents I really didn't want to go, but it soon became clear that once again I would not have a choice. They had planned a trip together and needed us to support them by staying in Selma.

I was petrified because this was happening, but it was inevitable. Two days later school had ended for the summer and we packed the car, and Mom kept trying to convince me I was going to have a great time. The only thing that kept me from running up the road screaming was the anticipation of seeing Nelly again.

The entire three hour drive from Mobile to Selma I prayed that we would have a car accident or my parents would have a change of heart. All I could do was stare out the back seat window up at the tops of the trees and try not to imagine what would be in store for me this summer.

I hope we don't have to start next year with one of those "what did you do for summer break presentations" at school. I would hate to let everyone know that I spent my summer trying to avoid being raped and beaten.

After we had arrived and my parents left we settled in with them, the routine was established quickly. Every evening, as soon as the dishes were done, I began to pace, straining my brain to find things to do. I would go to my friend's houses and invite myself to have dinner with them, stay out in the woods until after dark if possible. I knew I had to stay busy and out of my grandfather's reach. But I often couldn't escape his clutches.

He would ask me to come into his den and "talk" with him. He'd found a new game that gave him a lot of pleasure. Of course I didn't enjoy it at all.

It began with his evening cocktail, Cutty Sark and water. Mema began making them around six o'clock every evening and asked me to take the drink to Pop in the den. I would grab the thirty two ounce plastic glass feeling the condensation drip over my hands. I bitched the entire way as I walked across their mosaic grey tile kitchen floor to step down into the den. Every night, he'd insist I try some of his "real man's drink."

With my first sip I gagged and thought *it tastes like gasoline smells.*

It was awful. To this day, I can't tolerate drinking scotch. It burned all the way down my throat and the sickening aftertaste lingered in my mouth for hours. It tasted so awful that I always shudder when I had to drink it.

After that little ritual, he'd ask me to sit with him in his chair so he could play his twisted game. The brown vinyl recliner was large enough for the two of us to recline in comfortably. He set his scotch on the table beside it, sipping it occasionally. He always lured me into his chair by telling me it was the perfect place to see the television.

I'd rather have been reading, but if I refused, he always had an awful threat handy, something I was sure he would do, so I always gave in.

This was his sick way of creating the right atmosphere for a sexual encounter with him. As I crawled into his chair, my entire body would start shaking, *please let this chair fall apart, please let someone come down here and interrupt* I would think to myself as I literally hugged the arm of the brown vinyl praying that this time he'd leave me alone. I always held out the hope that he truly wanted me to sit and watch TV without any underlying selfish intentions.

Of course that never happened. The only times we did actually watch TV was when he was unexpectedly interrupted. While my parents were "saving their marriage," I spent evenings with this cruel ritual, wishing I was anywhere but here. Fortunately, having my sister along helped some. He couldn't be as free with me as he would have liked.

When the summer ended, I was ecstatic to be back in Mobile to start our new school year. The trip my parents took and their time away from us ultimately did not save their marriage. They were separated by the time I turned twelve years old, and eventually divorced. As their separation and divorce progressed, my sister became more and more rebellious.

She would wake me up at night to sleep in her bed so Mom and Dad would not know that she had sneaked out. They never checked on me after I went to bed, so she took advantage of that. She also made me her lookout on the way to school so she could slip into a cluster of trees and smoke. She may have made straight A's in school, but she was the devil's child at home.

We attended a Christian school, and I became immersed in religion. Though they taught us about God and sin, they never made the distinction of when you would go to hell. Every time I was the lookout for Evelyn's smoking ventures, I was convinced God would just send her to hell without giving me the opportunity to save her soul. I would pray *Lord, I know you made her smart but sometimes she does so many stupid things, please don't take her to hell, she can't seem to help it.*

The day I decided to save her soul I informed my mother that I needed to save my sister from the pits of hell. I told her everything I could possibly think of doing what I could to confess my sister's sins. My mom sat there and listened to every word I had to say and syllable by syllable her face became more and more red.

I was so relieved and certain I had redeemed Evelyn from her unimaginable fate. I couldn't wait to see the amazing transformation in her. I heard her voice as she walked up to our front door uttering words that were inaudible. Instead of walking through the front door with a beautiful halo and an aura of purity around her, Evelyn came in smelling like liquor.

She had a letter informing Mom that she had been suspended for being disrespectful to a teacher. The letter stated that my sister had "shot the bird" to her teacher Mrs. Hollingsworth.

Indeed, no good deed goes unpunished. I knew without a doubt that my parents would divorce now.

Dad has always worked very hard, putting work before family, which made me resent him. When my parents divorced, however, I realized it wasn't work that kept him away from us; it was what he had to deal with at home. I think he worked so many hours because the people he worked with knew him in a different way, and he could escape the emotional responsibilities of a high-maintenance wife, a rebellious daughter, and a son who apparently displeased him. At work, he was successful. At home, he failed miserably, and he was so competitive he chose to walk away rather than trying to fix what went wrong.

CHAPTER 4

Chaos And Loss

Following the divorce, in the middle of my seventh-grade year, my sister and I moved with my mother across the Mobile Bay to Lake Forest. Evelyn and I would travel back and forth to Mobile every day because we didn't want to have to start a new school mid-year and we could end the year at Independent Methodist School.

I became friends with people in Lake Forest who loved horses, and I spent the majority of my time there learning how to trust again.

I loved the horses. I really resonated with what they represented. Horses are magnificent creatures, and I have always enjoyed being around them. They are unconditionally accepting and even loving. Still, they are strong enough to take care of themselves.

I soon changed my focus from religion to horses, and the knowledge I gained from these amazing animals helped to set my course for life.

Horses have a way of teaching humans about boundaries in life. Walking behind one is ill-advised, because they may kick you. They establish a perimeter and typically do not allow their space to be invaded. That helped me understand that I needed to let people know what they could and could not do to me, which was empowering and strengthening, given my experiences.

While I was turning to horses to ease my pain during the divorce, my sister began to sink into alcohol. She continued to make poor choices with friends, drugs, and even stealing. She became a real headache for my mother.

With Mom struggling with the new found status of divorcée and Evelyn struggling with alcohol and drugs, I was determined to be the good child. I kept my behavior exemplary and tried to stay in the background. I really hated seeing someone as depressed as my mother was at that time.

As it turned out, Mom had an ulterior motive for moving to Lake Forest. She wanted to stay close to Dad, and try every ploy she could think of to win him back. She kept reminding him how weak she was and telling him how she needed him.

Her strategies accomplished nothing more than to create anger and unhappiness for her. One night I heard her throw the phone across her bedroom while screaming at my dad. I opened her bedroom door to check on her and found a woman who looked possessed, angry over not getting her way as she normally did. Her hair was matted, mascara ran down her face, and things were in disarray all over the room.

What has he done to her this time? "Mom, come on let's get up and get you in bed." She sobbed over my shoulder as I gently tucked her in bed for the night.

She tried presenting herself as a victim, and even managed to get her car stolen so my dad had to take her places. That plan utterly backfired on her, and we wound up walking for a few days until her car was miraculously found. She claimed she had gone to the grocery store but had forgotten and left her keys in the ignition. Ironically, the police were never involved.

I thought I would be at Daphne High School in Lake Forest for eighth grade, but that wasn't the case. Mom found out Dad had a girlfriend, and she decided to punish him by moving us back to Selma. I will never forget the day; it was as if a national disaster had happened , so burned is it in my memory. She slowly walked into my bedroom and sat down on the edge of my bed and said, "we are going to have to move back to Selma to live with Mema and Pop for a while because I am just not able to afford living here on my own."

"What about Dad, can't he give you the money we need?"

"No, and this is not a discussion. I just wanted to let you know. In the morning I need for you to start packing your things." She stood up quickly and looked around my room.

"What, why so soon, can't we finish out the summer here?" I sat up in the bed with such concern on my face with a begging tone.

"Please don't argue with me. Just wake up in the morning and start packing. I have some boxes you can use in the living room." She avoided eye contact, abruptly stood, and walked out of my room.

"Mom, please don't, I want to stay here, I am not trying to argue I just don't want to go back to Selma, please Mom!"

I was happy in Lake Forest because of the horses, friends and because I didn't have Dad putting me down every day or Pop abusing me.

I knew she wondered why I was so opposed to the idea, but I couldn't tell her I was afraid because Pop might kill her if we moved back to Selma. I knew she would never ask me why I was so opposed to the idea either because she wanted her way.

He had made the threat to kill my mother if I told his secrets so many times that I absolutely believed him. I thought the only way I could keep my mother safe was to keep her in another place, away from him.

After the night ended and I knew I had no choice in the decision, I had to step up and be brave.

"Mom, I am sorry for the way I acted last night and I will be okay going back to Selma if we don't have to live with Mema and Pop."

"I promise we will have our own home."

She did keep her promise but what she failed to tell me at that point was that they would be caring for me almost all the time so she could go out with friends and enjoy her pity parties.

Once my parents divorced, I saw very little of my dad, and he was only mentioned when he was alleged to have visited some terrible act upon my mother. Though he was never around, he and my mother continued to fight about money. When she found out Dad had a new girlfriend, she became convinced that was where all of Dad's money was going.

She began telling Dad she needed to rent a different house and needed money for the deposit and the first- and last-month's rent. She also said she didn't have enough money for me to go to Morgan Academy, which was where I attended school when we'd live in Selma previously.

"What do you mean I can't go to Morgan Academy? That is where all of my friends are"

I begged her to find a way because it meant I'd have to go to Westside Middle School. It had a horrible reputation for violence and drug use. Evelyn was attending Selma High School, which had the same type of atmosphere, and this was her senior year.

Even with all of the begging, I could muster up it didn't work. I still had to go to Westside Middle School, which was my first time ever going to a public school.

My first day of class, I walked though the huge front double doors and as I crossed the threshold I was engulfed by the smell of mildew and pubescence. The air was stale and musty, as if the school had been shut up for years. People were wandering the halls and everyone was so loud. I made my way down a long hallway and found a room that I thought would look in some way different on the inside. I found my desk and started my prayers again. Eventually my homeroom teacher walked in, took roll, and left. While he was out of the room, two guys were rolling joints and another guy named Rabbit lit one. I was clearly out of my element and scared to death.

Panicked, I thought to myself, *okay, just lean back in the desk and act as if you don't care about anything, cross your arms and keep your head focused on the desktop.* I felt as if I was acting like someone on a television show trying to "be cool" and unknowingly making a huge, social-misfit fool of myself.

School had always been a sanctuary for me, but it wouldn't be that way this year, I could just feel it.

At Westside Middle School, I became an expert on skipping class. I was dropped off at the front door by Evelyn, and would walk through the school holding my breath because of the terrible moldy odor, down the back steps, and spend the day hiding in the shrubs at the back of the school. I had my lunch with me so I didn't have to worry about missing a meal or going to the cafeteria. I did this two to three times a week, and my grades never suffered because my previous education was much more advanced than what Westside offered.

Mom was completely wrapped up in herself. She didn't care about our schools or anything. She actually enjoyed making Dad feel guilty about the awful schools we attended. She never seemed to notice that Evelyn and I were struggling with making friends at school or anywhere else.

I kept in touch with Mema and Pop, not because of them, but as a way of staying in touch with Nelly. When I would get home from school I would walk into the house and call her. More often than not when I asked to speak with her, Mema said no. She always used the same excuse every time, "She is working and can't come to the phone."

Every day I went home and begged my mother to send me to another school. She told me Dad wasn't giving her enough child support to pay for it, and I should talk to him about it.

My days were horror-filled at school. A boy was stabbed in the bathroom; two pregnant girls were fighting because they were pregnant by the same eighth grader. The fight ended with one of the girls lying lifeless at the bottom of the stairs, after being thrown down by her opponent.

After my incident with Dirk and spending the summer with Mema and Pop, I became indifferent and numb to everything. I didn't care whether people liked me or not. I still missed Nelly; nothing could change that. But Mom was in the throes of a divorce, and her children were relegated to a lower place in her list of priorities.

I became friends with a classmate, Jessica, who was a neighbor and had horses. That's when I reconnected with these majestic animals more deeply than anything I had ever experienced in Lake Forest. It was a good exercise because I wasn't just learning to trust people again; I was simply learning how to trust.

I began to beg for a horse of my own, and I did everything I could do to wear Dad down. Eventually, to my disbelief, he finally promised to buy me a horse. The only catch was that I had to find an affordable place to board it. I already had a place in mind. I went to visit Jessica and explained to her parents what Dad had said.

I pleaded my case, "I promise that I will be here every day to clean out the stalls and do whatever work you need me to do in exchange for rent."

Her dad said," I will do this on one condition; I need for you to be here every day before school and on the weekends to help me around here." I couldn't believe he was willing to do this. I was elated beyond words and just jumped up and hugged him. "Thank you so much, you have no idea what this means to me. I will not let you down."

They knew that Mom and Dad had their issues and they also knew how passionate I was with their horses. The next day I met with Dad and this time he had no excuses left. He finally broke down and bought a beautiful chestnut Tennessee Walker named Charlie.

I kept my promise to her parents just as they kept their promise to me. This time, the knowledge I gained about horses in Lake Forest was something I could relate to myself. They represented what I wanted to be – strong, loving, powerful, and able to take care of myself. I also wanted to be the kind of person who loved like they did, unconditionally, but with the right boundaries.

I now knew that I needed to create these same types of boundaries for myself. I just had to learn to do it in a way that made sense. I felt this realization meant I was getting healthy again and putting things in order for myself. I found a kind of peace I had not known before.

However, my world would once again become interrupted with a horrific event.

I got out of school one day and found Pop waiting for me. He said Mom had suffered a stroke and the right side of her face was paralyzed. I had no idea what he was talking about, *she is only thirty two years old and I thought strokes only happened to old people.*

When we got home, my mom was surrounded by a group of people and looked like she was very happy. Based on the description Pop gave me I expected to see her cheek hanging down to her shoulder with drool coming out of her mouth. I went running over to see her; I saw very little wrong with her face.

As usual, he loves playing these sick games with me to keep me in fear. I knew she wouldn't look that bad.

I visited Dad that weekend for the first time in months. I told him about Mom's stroke, and all he said was, "I hope she doesn't use it as a crutch to be manipulative."

I was confused, telling him she didn't need crutches. He explained what his statement meant, and I realized it could be true.

On Mom's side of the family I was closest to Mark and Nicole, who were my favorite cousins, and the children of Uncle Lance, my mother's brother, and Aunt Janice.

Mark and I were more like brothers. He and Nelly were the two people who helped me keep my sanity when Pop was abusing me. Nicole is his older sister, and she is still one of the most beautiful women I've ever known. She looks like a perfectly drawn doll with soft golden curls and was graced by God with intelligence, humor, talent, and compassion.

Growing up she and I were not close, but as adults, we've reached out to each other and now we are practically inseparable. She has become my confidant and soul mate and has supported me through the roughest decisions and situations in my life. She is an independent thinker and an achiever, knowing exactly what she needs to do to get to the next level in her life. She has been my only good link with my family because of her acceptance of me for who I am. She saves judgment for God and embraces people that many would turn away from because she looks at their souls, not just what's on the outside.

Mark and I were only months apart in age, so it seemed natural that we would be best friends and do everything together. A lot of people didn't appreciate Mark because he was hyperactive. He would bounce from one subject to the next, and then punch you in the stomach and laugh without a thought.

What people did not see was how big his heart was. We frequently spent the night at each other's houses, and would talk for hours about anything and everything. Our conversations centered on our two passions—horses for me and motorcycles for him. We were different enough to appreciate each other and alike enough to fight like brothers.

We were both good at what we did. I was Southeastern Junior Champ Barrel Racer, and Mark was a dirt bike motorcycle racer. He could jump hills and do stunts and was just generally very impressive on a motorcycle.

We became very close that summer of my eighth grade year. I think a lot of it had to do with experiencing puberty together. He was becoming a good-looking guy and an independent thinker like Nicole. He didn't worry about peer pressure and paved his own way in the world.

He and I had both been through a lot of tough times. I had gone through the anxiety of my parents' divorce, and he had some physical problems that were somewhat mysterious in nature. He suffered a grand mal seizure when he was eight years old and had never had any problems like that before. He immediately went into a coma and was in the hospital for weeks and was even taken to a larger city. He eventually recovered without any adverse effects.

We were both growing up becoming responsible young adults, to the relief of all our parents.

One of our favorite activities was to camp out in my grandparents' backyard. We enjoyed it because it felt like we were away from everybody and on our own. We could smell the aroma produced from the sap of the Pecan trees and hear the crickets having their beautiful evening symphony. It was so peaceful. We'd pretend we were in the middle of a forest and had to protect ourselves, hunt for food, and protect each other. We made up all kinds of games and just had a great time together.

One night, I decided it was time to ask Mark a very important question. We were lying with our heads outside the tent's zipper door so we could look up at the stars. I gathered up my courage and said, "Hey, Mark, can I ask you a question?"

Without moving his gaze from the sky he said, "Yep."

My heart was thumping because my biggest fear was he would look at me differently if he knew the truth.

I quickly asked, "Has anyone ever done anything to you they shouldn't have?"

"At school, this kid tried to blame me for something I didn't do, and I got in trouble for it anyway," he said.

I wasn't surprised about that. Mark was always in some type of trouble. He was the greatest kid, but he was so hyperactive he was always getting into messes. He had a pretty bad reputation at school. That was part of his charm to me, though; I enjoyed him for who he was.

That comment didn't help me, so I decided to ask him point blank. Keeping my eyes on the evening stars, I said, "Has anyone ever touched your private parts?"

Unexpectedly he turned the tables on me. "Why? Has anyone ever touched you in your private parts?"

I panicked and didn't know what to say. Finally, I mumbled, "Maybe."

Mark was a rebel at heart and really didn't care about hurting anyone's feelings. I knew he would tell me the truth because we were so close. He said, "Well, yeah, Pop did, but only once."

I jerked around to look at him and asked, "What did you do?"

He faced me and said, "What choice did I have?"

Since he had confided in me, I felt compelled to be honest with him. When I gave him some of the details, he looked at me and said, "But it only happened once, right?"

I was embarrassed for him to know the whole truth, so I just returned my gaze to the sky and said, "Oh, yeah, only once." As the lie crossed my lips, I briefly wondered why it happened to me more than it had to Mark.

The old man thought he was sly. I guess he never figured out that we knew the sound of his footsteps when he went wandering around during the night. We heard the sliding door open, and we took off, running away from him as fast as we could. The good thing about being outside when it was dark was we could get away fast, and he couldn't find us.

Mark and I always made big plans for the weekends. Our houses were only blocks from each other, and we were together as often as we could, even on school nights.

This particular weekend we were celebrating his birthday by going skating with our girlfriends. I had turned thirteen in September, and now it was November and Mark's turn to become a teenager.

We were finishing lunch with Nelly at my grandparent's house while we planned our skating adventure. Nelly asked, "Now, are you boys going to treat those girls nice?"

"Of course we are Nelly, as long as they pay their own way!"

She looked at me and started laughing. "Now you know, when you start courting young ladies, there is a lot of responsibility you will take on, like paying for everything."

Abruptly our conversation ended because Evelyn came in and fussed at Mark for riding his motorcycle to Mema and Pops' house.

"Well, he rode Charlie and we have been out riding on the dirt roads together." He wasn't old enough to be on the main roads and came through the back lanes and side roads. Finally, Evelyn offered to follow him home to be sure he made it back to his house alright.

As I rode my beautiful horse toward the barn, I thought about how perfect my life was now that Mark and I could be together so much. He was like a brother to me. He even made the abuse I experienced from my grandfather that summer easier to bear. Spending time with Mark was worth everything.

Buying Charlie was probably the nicest thing my father had ever done for me. In my heart, I knew Dad only bought Charlie because he was guilty about divorcing Mom and being away from me. In reality, I didn't care about that too much. I loved Charlie, and there wasn't any better place to be in the world at that moment.

I kept Charlie in an old barn that had formerly been used for dairy cattle. It was an interesting place, and I loved being there. It was near Mema and Pops' home. The barn was at the end of a long dirt road, close to our house. The white of the barn was a stark contrast to the red clay around it and the lush green leaves on the trees above it. It smelled like hay, molasses and honeysuckle all rolled into one odor that was simply indescribably amazing. It was in a wooded area, and my legs were always covered with scratches because I'd scrape against bushes and trees on the way to the barn.

While I was getting Charlie settled in his stall for the night, I heard what sounded like an explosion in the quiet of the barn.

That was unusual.

My stomach tightened immediately. I knew something had occurred, but I had no idea what. I kept thinking somebody would come and tell me what had happened.

When I finished, I walked to the end of the dirt road that led to the barn, waiting to be picked up. I felt panicked but I could not understand why. When no one came, I ran to Griffin's Grocery Store to use their phone. I burst through the door smelling of sweat and horses and yelled "can I call

Mema to see if she knows what was going on?" I just assumed Mr. Griffin would know what I was talking about since he has known me my entire life.

"Sure. I heard the loud noise also," he said as he placed the phone on the counter. I dialed the phone and almost immediately Mema picked up and said, "Mark has been in a terrible accident. You need to get home right now!"

"What happened to Mark?" I yelled into the phone, but she had already hung up.

"Is everything okay?" Mr. Griffin asked looking concerned. "Can I take you somewhere?"

I replied in a panic stricken voice, "I don't know, I don't know what is happening, thank you for letting me use your phone."

The fear in my gut told me something bad had happened to Mark. I hurried back to the dirt road, and finally Nicole and her boyfriend Tommy picked me up. When I asked about Mark, Nicole roughly shoved me into the back seat and said, "Just get in the car now."

When they headed toward Mema and Pops' house I said, "Where are you going? I'm supposed to meet Mark at your house."

Nicole was very upset and crying so very hard. She turned and said, "That isn't going to happen, because Mark had a wreck on the way to our house. We have to go to Mema and Pop's to find out what is going on."

Everyone in my family, except Mark's parents, was there when we arrived. I kept going from person to person, asking what had happened, but nobody would tell me anything. I guess they thought I was too young to understand. Finally, Nelly pulled me aside and told me about the accident.

"Mark was on his way to put up his motorcycle and Evelyn was following him when a big truck ran right into the side of him."

"Do you know if he is going to be alright?"

It turned out the adults were right, it *was* difficult for me to understand what exactly happened. Apparently, a power company truck, being driven by a man who had been working for twenty-four hours without a break, turned in front of Mark. He said he hadn't seen Mark coming toward him. Mark slammed into the side of the truck. He was so close to home that his house could be seen from the site of the accident.

Evelyn was following right behind him and saw what happened and hurried out to help as much as she could. She told me his head began swelling immediately and all she was able to do was keep him stable until help came.

58

Every day I asked to go see Mark, but my family wouldn't let me. I cried every night, fearing my best friend was going die. I spent hours talking to Nelly about Mark, trying to make sense of it. To comfort me, she always said, "God needs angels."

When Dad and I were in the chapel at the hospital, his only words of comfort were for himself as he said, "I'm glad it was him and not you."

I looked at him in disbelief, stunned he would say that. *Are you crazy,* I thought to myself, *I wish it were me and not him.* Still, I knew for my dad, it was truly an emotional outburst.

After six weeks on life support, Mark died. They told me his blood became too thick to circulate through his body, and his brain suffocated. That never made sense to me, so I feared they were mad at us and didn't want us to talk anymore because Mark had told them his dirty secret that I also held private about Pop.

Even when it was time for Mark's funeral, I couldn't accept that he was dead. I was convinced it was a conspiracy by my family to keep him and me apart. I kept promising that Mark and I would separate if they'd just let me know he was alive and well.

I guess my pleas got to them because they finally decided to open the coffin for me. They told me his face had been hurt badly in the accident and he was almost unrecognizable. When they raised the lid, I realized how right they were. The face on the person in the coffin looked somewhat like Mark, but was much larger than I remembered. Mark's lips were laced together with thick strands of black thread, and they were huge.

Accepting there was nothing more I could do for Mark, I went to the gravesite service and watched in horror as the casket, with my beloved cousin inside, was lowered into the ground. We then went to a memorial service at First Independent Protestant Church that was packed with hundreds of people showing their support and respect for my family.

By the time everything was done, it was late evening, and I was emotionless and exhausted. I thought I'd be leaving the funeral with Mom and Dad or my aunt and my sister. Instead, Pop volunteered to take me home. I was too numb to care. I just wanted to go home and grieve.

He drove around behind the church, where there was a dirt road that was a shortcut to their house. I was just staring up at the sky, trying to find the angel God needed and wondering why he took my angel from me.

God, don't you know he was the only person who loved me and you took him away? I know you need angels but I needed him I am certain more than you. How can you do this to me and my life, what do you want from me? What do I need to do to have you love me and keep the people that love me in my life? First, Mom and Dad divorce and now Mark is gone from me too.

I was so deep in thought I didn't even realize the car had stopped and Pop was quietly looking at me.

He stroked my hair, with his left hand propped on the steering wheel. Then he unzipped his pants and told me he knew what would make me feel better.

My stomach contents were in my throat and I fought not to throw up. When I told him I wasn't going to do it, he hit me in the back of the head. I could feel the power of his blow all the way into my teeth.

"You don't have a choice," he said coldly.

"You can't make my choices," I said frustrated and wanting to maintain some type of dignity during the funeral. "I make them."

"The decision's been made," he said, and pushed my head toward his crotch.

As he pulled me closer, I thought *maybe this was why God took Mark. He didn't want Mark to go through what I was and he could protect him better in heaven.* It made sense to me that the only protection from his abuse was death.

As my face made contact with skin I could smell his rancid odor, I slid over to the passenger door. As my hand reached the door handle, he yanked the back of my shirt. Putting all his weight on my shoulders so I couldn't move, he grabbed my belt to undo my pants.

"Please don't do this to me, not today, please not today," I begged, which seemed to make him more violent. In disbelief that he would choose a day like today, I fought as hard as I could.

I kicked, punched, and did everything I knew to do, but he was so big that he easily moved his body between my legs. He placed his hands in the middle of my back and forced my rear end up into the air. With one forcible thrust, he shoved himself inside me. The pain was unimaginable. I could feel my skin rip and tear and every muscle I had clinched up as tight as it could to prevent him from being able to continue, but the more I fought the more intense the pain became. I could feel the blood start to trickle down the inside of my thigh. It was all too much for my little body to handle.

I knew I couldn't fight anymore so I became limp and catatonic. I could feel myself slip into a state of unconsciousness. I focused on the most wonderful thing I could think about at that moment *Nelly, please talk to me about anything I can't take this anymore.* I could see her face and hear her laughter and that was all I could make out before he brutally brought me back to reality.

He smashed my face against the passenger window. Expecting to feel pain, I felt nothing. It was as if my soul had left my body and I was witnessing this from the outside. I remember seeing the church steeple in the distance and silently said, *Thank you, God, for taking Mark away from all this. When will you take me?*

He finished and pushed me to make sure I was listening to him as he demanded I put my pants on. I slowly moved and started to pull my pants up from around my ankles and noticed blood on the seat from where he had raped me. I pulled up one pants leg at a time and loosely tried to tuck in my shirt. Starring into space, feeling the blood and semen ooze out of me, I just so wished that death had come to me and not to Mark.

When we arrived at my aunt and uncle's house I saw all of the people that had come back to their house from the church. I was absorbed into the background because everyone else was so focused on Mark being gone. My shirt was partially un-tucked, my pants had dried blood on them and my hair was uncharacteristically disheveled. I had a huge lump on my head from where it had been shoved into the window but the room was so dimly lit it was able to go unnoticed.

I lowered my head hoping to be invisible by all and went straight to Mark's bedroom, pushing what had happened into the darkest recesses of my mind. My head hurt and my rear end was still bleeding, and all I could do was sit in Mark's beanbag chair and beg him to come back home. I fell asleep in the chair, and I swear I remember Mark coming down to me to let me know he would be there when I needed him.

He didn't appear as a solid object, just as a light, a beautiful, warm yellow light.

CHAPTER 5

SURVIVING THE SEAS

W hen the school year ended, Mom said we were going to move in with Mema and Pop. Evelyn was moving back to Mobile when she graduated to live with Dad, and Mom was concerned because she was losing her portion of child-support money. That made her feel it was necessary for us to live with Mema and Pop.

I reminded her of the conversation we had in Lake Forest. She had promised that we wouldn't have to live with them when we moved back to Selma. She said everything was planned, and she was only able to get out of her lease because of her stroke. She wanted to go ahead and move so she wouldn't have to work for a while.

Dad was right; Mom was using her stroke as a crutch to get exactly what she wanted. She was telling me that she would not be able to get a job "with her face looking like it did," even though it was hardly noticeable. I knew that wasn't the case. I had seen all types of people working before, and many of them were truly disfigured, burned or even wheelchair-bound. This was not something that would keep her from being employed, but instead it would keep her where she was comfortable: in the victim role.

Once we moved in with Mema and Pop, they rallied around Mom and were very supportive. We received such a warm welcome that I began to think the abuse was over. Hopefully, they'd focus all their energy on helping her. This was not to be the case.

One afternoon Pop had me out working on one of his cars, which was something I truly hated doing. He would go to auto auctions and buy cars that were wrecked or damaged, at ridiculously low prices, then repair them like they were new and sell them for a significant profit. He was certainly talented when it came to understanding engine mechanics, which made him very successful.

He started his own car lot, but never had more than one or two cars to sell at a time. He would place them for sale in the front yard so people could see them when they drove past. His reputation also kept him in business. He was a member of many of the associations in town like the Lions Club and The Masons, which is where most of his reputation was built. These groups were incredibly secretive, especially pertaining to any members who had achieved status within the organization.

On this particular day, he was working on an old Saab and he was trying to get the engine to start. I had no idea about cars and had even less of an interest in their mechanical workings. I would just sit there while he was working on them just to hand him tools, usually fantasizing about being anywhere else. For some time, his disposition seemed a bit off. He was being more degrading than usual and I could not figure out what to do.

If I just stand here he will tell me I am lazy, if I start to hand him tools and they are the wrong ones then I will be stupid, so the best thing I can do is wait until the next order is placed. I wish I could just walk away, but if I did that I know he will kill me.

The next order came more quickly than I thought. I was looking at different tools trying to anticipate his next need. Out of the blue came a command I had not heard before and it alarmed me. I was sitting beside the front wheel on the ground with my arms on my knees and my head resting on my forearms. He was bent over the fender looking under the hood struggling trying to figure out what the issue seemed to be.

I heard a hissing sound like an aerosol can being sprayed. Then he backed out from under the hood, "put you face close to the engine and tell me if there is a spark when I turn the engine over," he barked. His tone was not really mean but more sinister than I had ever heard before. Not really sure what to do I turned and slowly looked up at him.

"Why do I need to do that? Can't you just turn the key and hear if the engine will start or not?" With one swift yank he grabbed me by my hair and pulled me up so quickly that I was on my feet before I realized what had happened. I was frightened, and I knew this was not the time to question him.

"Now, like I just told you, put your face right here and tell me if you see a spark." He grabbed me by my head and positioned my face exactly where he wanted it to be. When he walked away I moved my face and put it down closer to the engine. I could not make out the odor that I smelled. I recognized the scent of oil and gas but there was another odor that smelled like alcohol mixed with lighter fluid.

"Are you exactly where I told you to be?" I didn't want him to know that I had moved my head a little bit because the fumes of whatever it was that he had sprayed were burning my eyes.

"Yes, I am right where you told me to be." I thought that I would be able to see the spark but more than that I knew that the engine was either going to start or not. Either way that would determine if there was a spark. He hesitated for a brief second and then yelled, "Okay here I go."

Following those words it was as if it were in slow motion. I heard the car key turn and then I saw the spark and within less than a second, a flame came shooting up out of the engine right where he had sprayed. Before I had the chance to react I could feel my head getting incredibly hot. I could smell my hair burning. What he had sprayed on the engine was ether. When it sparked, a flame shot up and caught my hair on fire.

I panicked and quickly remembered that while I was sitting by the front tire I was looking at the water in Lucky's dog bowl. I immediately went running to the dish and shoved my head into it while he laughed and laughed. I could hear the sizzle of the water retarding the flames that were shooting up from my head and I was splashing water all over the back of my neck. I could smell the disgusting odor of burnt and wet hair. I was terrified to take my head out of the water because I was not sure if the flames were out.

I cautiously stuck my hands into the bowl and touched my head. There was hardly any hair left and all I could feel was fuzz in some places and strands of hair in other. It was obvious that this had caused damage but I was so glad I had moved my face. Exactly where the flames shot up is where my face was positioned. He was truly trying to kill me. I was infuriated.

I said, "You almost burned my face off!"

He replied, "That'll make a man out of you."

I was so surprised that someone trying to catch me on fire was a path to manhood.

"No, that is what will kill me," I said with fury.

I went running in the house and looked in the mirror. Most of my hair had been burned to the scalp and I had some redness in the very front of my hairline near my forehead.

What a freak, he is truly crazy and has no regard for anyone. How am I going to start school next week looking like this? I was so upset that I took out the clippers that Mema kept in her cabinet and cut the rest off so that I could get rid of that singed hair odor.

The next week came and I was so excited and anxious. I was finally leaving Westside Middle School and going back to Morgan Academy. I had been at Morgan for my first through fifth grades, and I was eager to be around my old friends, to see how they had changed and grown. I noticed immediately that all my friends seemed different. I couldn't tell if it were because it looked like I had just gotten over lice or recently been released from a concentration camp thanks to Pop's antics from the prior week or if it were me.

I'd been gone so long that they had formed new cliques and I was finding it hard to re-connect with anyone. I would try and sit beside them at lunch and they would move to the other table, I tried speaking to them in the hallways and they would not speak back and completely ignored me as if I were not even there. I even tried sitting beside them in different classes and they would literally pick up their things and move to the other side of the class room.

Even my cousin treated me differently. I had tried so hard to get back in my circle but it seemed like I was the only one interested. Mom and Dad were now divorced and none of their parents were. Mom attributed their not liking me to her divorce. I didn't agree; something was different.

They all sensed that I had changed. I knew I had as well. I was not as jovial as I had been before. I was different and I knew it but I couldn't be anyone other than myself. Occasionally, when no one else was around, one of them would speak to me but nothing else. There was also a new sport in school–picking on me because I was different.

On Labor Day at Morgan Academy, we could buy flowers and put an anonymous note on them to give to other students. It was the perfect way to get the school ready for the annual Sadie Hawkins dance that normally kicked off the events for the school year. The proceeds from this went to charity. I received a carnation, and I thought it was from my only friend, Jennifer, who shared my love of horses. The card read, "I love you, and I think you're sexy."

I was so excited because it signaled to me that I was being accepted, and I quickly went to find Jennifer and asked if she'd given it to me. She looked at me perplexed and wanted to say yes at first but stuttered, "No, uh, no sorry I really didn't."

I was confused because of everyone there she was the only person who was even likely to think of me in this way. About that time, it was revealed who the true sender was. Al, one of the guys who was a good friend when I'd been at the school previously came running over to me and looked over my shoulder, "What does the card say?" his sarcasm was clear.

He ripped the flower from my hand and loudly read the card, "I love you, and I think you're sexy." He puckered his lips, faked kisses at me then turned and looked at all of his friends standing in the hallway laughing at me.

I felt like a complete fool and a stranger among friends I thought I could trust. I was so mad, but I had to find a way to regain my dignity. I had been through enough exercises to understand the passage to manhood, and I thought it was time to teach Al one of the lessons I had learned. I had always been an easy going kid and put up with a lot but I had finally had it.

Later that day, I gave him a little present of my own. After the final bell had rung I waited for him to round the corner to go to his locker. I stopped him and said,

"I think what you did was one of the most horrible things a friend has ever done to me."

He dismissively remarked, "Who said you were my friend? Just because I knew you in elementary school certainly doesn't mean I like you today. You are poor white trash and the only reason you go to this school is because of your grandparents."

I couldn't hold back, everything around me started to get dark and the next thing I knew I had him pinned up against the locker and I was pounding on his face. I took him by his head and shoved him into the locker. He started to put his hands up in front of his face and I grabbed him by his wrist and pushed him onto the ground and started kicking and punching at anything I could come in contact with. All I could see was blood and darkness and then I felt arms all around me pulling me off of him. The physical education teacher, science teacher and Assistant Principal were all there trying to get me to stop. They called the school nurse to look him over and pulled both of us into the office.

Fortunately for me he had a reputation as being a trouble maker and I did not, so the school principal knew he had done something to instigate the fight. I explained my side of the story and he lied about his. We were both suspended because I had participated in the fight and I could have walked away, but instead I chose to confront him at his locker.

We both insincerely apologized to each other just to get out of the principal's office, but things were never the same. He never bothered me to my face, but after that, he and some of his friends began calling Mema to tell her I was a "fag" and a "nigger lover," which made things even more horrifying at home. I would get home from school and Pop would ask me if I had any new "nigger boyfriends." I couldn't believe that they believed the boys at school.

I felt like there was no place I could go where people liked me for being me. I didn't know what a fag was and I certainly didn't take offense to being in love with anyone in the African-American race because that was the only place I felt loved. Nelly never judged me like my family did, so every day after school, instead of coming home to my family to tell them about my day, I would sneak and find Nelly and hide for the rest of the night talking with her until she left.

It was horrible to discover my "safe place" was no longer a comfort zone. I had all this going on at school and Pop's abuse at home. He was determined to "make me a man," which became his catch phrase. Little did he know I was more of a man than he would ever be.

Mom attributed my recent behavior at school to a lack of positive male influence since Dad was no longer around. Granted, when he was around, not all of his influence was necessarily positive.

There was a hurricane headed to the gulf, and Pop was moving his boat from Gulf Shores to Selma. During Hurricane Frederick we sustained so much damage, he was trying to take all precautions into consideration. Once he told everyone of his plan, he and Mom came up with the brilliant idea that this could be the male bonding that she felt I needed. I came home from school and about three hours later, when Mom came in from work, she pulled me into her bedroom to break the big news. "Guess what Pop and I have decided to do?" She was excited and her behavior seemed to be that of someone that had just solved a major life crisis.

"What?"

"You know that hurricane season seems to be going much later into the year than normal with the development of Hurricane Dennis?"

Still trying to understand the message I perplexingly partnered with her story. "Yes, I know that you all have been talking about it, why?"

"Well, with your father not being around, we thought it would be a great idea for you to go with Pop when he moves his boat from Gulf Shores to Selma to experience some male bonding."

Being only thirteen, I really didn't care about bonding with anyone especially him. "What about school?" Not that I really cared about school but the thought of being stuck on a boat with just the two of us started to worry me.

"I called the school today during my lunch hour and worked everything out. I will check you out of school early so you can join them." I didn't know what to say, it was obvious that the plans were made without my input as usual. Pop and I were going to meet his brother, Eddie, in Gulf Shores, and the three of us would bring the boat to Selma.

Sounding as if she had already counted on every counter objection I could think of I didn't see any other choice so I, feeling forced said "Okay when are we supposed to leave?" *Hopefully between now and whatever date she gives me I can come up with some type of excuse to get out of going.*

"I talked with the school and I will be checking you out tomorrow after lunch."

"Tomorrow, I have too much going on tomorrow! I have a science test and I wanted to spend some time with Charlie."

I can't come up with anything believable by tomorrow. Maybe if I fake an illness or something that will get me out of going. That had never worked in the past because Mom had the doctor on speed dial because of her illnesses and she could get me in first thing in the morning, medicated and ready to go by the afternoon.

With a conclusive tone, she looked at me and said, "You are going young man and that is the end of it. Why are you so bothered by it? Did you ever stop to think it could be fun?" Fun was the last thought I had about this trip, I was terrified and panicked.

Trying to get the last word in I forced a rebuttal with compassion, "I appreciate your concern for my lack of male companionship, but I really don't want to go." She thought I wanted to stay because of her needing me. In truth, she was immersed in her own issues and wasn't capable of good judgment for me.

I had lost the discussion and the next day she checked me out of school. She made it a point to go into the principal's office and brag about the boat trip being a great educational experience. A teacher's aide came to let me know she was waiting for me in the front office. I stalled as long as I could, begrudgingly walked up to the glass door, and put my hand on the cool metal handle. When I swung the door open I could smell her perfume lingering in the air so I knew she was there and that I was stuck going on this trip. She came from around the corner where she had been talking and looked at me, "Do you have everything?"

"I guess so. I am coming back, right?" I didn't know if she had different plans for me or not since she had already contemplated this trip without my knowledge.

She looked around the school office with a countenance of pure innocence. She walked over to me and put her hand on my shoulder and did her typical performance, especially now that she had a captive audience. "Oh, sweet son, I know you have been through so much with your Dad leaving us and all, but don't worry, you are never going anywhere without me." She slowly looked over her shoulder to check to see if her audience was paying attention, and put her arm around me as we walked out of the door. Immediately after the door shut behind us her attitude changed.

"What took you so long to get all of your things? Don't you know that they are waiting on you to go? I have packed everything I think you will need so when you get home you need to use the bathroom and jump right in the car." Feeling more like she was trying to get rid of me instead of do what was best for me I opened my car door and sarcastically gave my frustrated answer. "Fine, Okay."

Once we got home, I did as instructed and put my things into Pops car and ran inside to use the restroom. I rounded the corner and to my surprise Nelly was standing right there at the entrance way of the kitchen. "Nelly, I am sorry I didn't see you there." I had run right into her like a typical clumsy kid. She immediately grabbed me and pulled me into her body. I took a deep breath and could smell the aroma of the cocoa butter lotion that she used on her skin. "Little boy, you don't worry about anything. I know you are going to be just fine on this trip and I will be here as soon as you get back."

She pushed me back to look into my eyes and she didn't need to say another word. I knew she was scared for me and wanted nothing more than either to go with me or to help me come up with a reason not to go. "I love you, Nelly." She pulled me back and gingerly said "I love you too," just audible enough for only me to hear.

We loaded up the car and I jumped into the back seat, getting settled for the four hour drive. Pop had Uncle Lance drive us down to Gulf Shores. Pop wanted to drive his boat back to Selma, away from the risk of being damaged by the possible hurricane. I was excited to get to Gulf Shores because being there brought me many great memories.

Mema and Pop had a beach house in Gulf Shores, where we spent the majority of summers. It wasn't anything over the top, but it was a great little cabin. Made of cinderblock, it had three bedrooms and was right across the street from the bay. It had a huge kitchen, big enough to hold a picnic table for eight. One of the bedrooms was so large it had four queen-sized beds in it.

On most days, we would take the boat out into the ocean and dive off the top. It was intimidating to look at the water so far below, but once I jumped, it felt like I was flying until I hit the water where gentle arms of the ocean caught me and held on till I made it to the surface. I positively loved being in the water.

We also did a lot of deep sea fishing, and it always felt safe because everyone was there together. This seemed to be the only place that, as a family, we all got along. All of us cousins spent our days swimming, diving, fishing, and generally having fun on the beach. Undoubtedly, this trip would be much different. I just didn't know how different.

We arrived at the dock in Gulf Shores, and Uncle Eddie was standing there drinking, which was his normal activity. He had gotten a ride from a friend, and they had beaten us there by a day. He was a great guy, but had lost his wife to cancer a few years prior. Since her death, he had done nothing but drink to the point of passing out to cope with his loss. Uncle Lance and I dropped off Pop so he could get the boat ready for the trip to Selma, and we left for the store to buy some supplies.

When we got back to the docks, Pop seemed unusually quiet and kept talking about being concerned about the engine room. *Oh, great does this mean we don't have to go on the trip?* Not really paying attention, I loaded the supplies we had just purchased down stairs in the cabin.

The boat was beautiful. Made from imported mahogany, its beautifully stained body was about forty feet long. It was accentuated by beautiful stainless steel handrails and intricate nautical silver inlays on the floor and walls. There was a door beside the captain's chair that led down into the cabin area of the boat. Once the door was opened it revealed three steps that led down to a fully equipped kitchen including a stove, refrigerator, and sink.

Beside the kitchen was the dining room table that could seat four people comfortably. It also folded down into a nice sized bed. Across from the dining room table was a couch that could be converted into bunk beds. They were comfortable to sleep on, but they had absorbed so much moisture they had a hint of mold in the fabric, as did the rest of the cabin area. Before the couch to the right of the entry door was the bathroom that included a toilet, sink and shower.

Beyond the dining room table and the couch at the hull of the cabin where the boats bow came to a point was a large area full of cushions. The royal blue cushions were surrounded by the most beautiful deep wood color walls that were perfectly crafted to curve to the shape of the boat. The silver inlays that surrounded the lights were simply mesmerizing.

It was a private area, separates from the rest of the cabin by a curtain that could be snapped to the wall. This area is where I typically preferred to sleep, because it was not easy to climb into and I felt somewhat secure. I would lie on the cushions at night and look up through the manhole that was at the top of this area and just stare at the stars.

Pop loved his boat and catered to its every need. He named it Novella, which I loved because it so closely resembled Nelly.

The engine room was below the gleaming deck, which was stained deep cherry red and trimmed in stainless steel. Nautical markings were around the edges. To get to the engine room, you had to pull up on these two silver loops that would lift the floor up to expose the ladder leading to the engines. After lifting the heavy floor boards, they could be secured so they wouldn't fall shut. I personally hated going down there because it smelled like a gas station garage and was an inferno with the noise level of a NASCAR track.

We cast off in the afternoon of the first day, and the later it got, the more Uncle Eddie drank. We all knew he was an alcoholic, so seeing him intoxicated was nothing new. He would walk around the deck and repeat the same conversation multiple times. If he cornered you long enough, he would tell you how much he loved you and then proceed on to a joke he has told a million times. I just avoided him.

As we got farther and farther away from land, the reality started to settle in on how vulnerable I was. I was limited with where I could go and hide from him, and I became more and more nervous. Pop was very quiet and intense. I knew in my gut something was going to happen, but I didn't know what. Frankly, I was really afraid he would throw me overboard, and tell Mom I jumped in and they couldn't find me. Actually, it would have been a better trip if that had happened.

Pop did the navigating, and he moved along smoothly in the crisp ocean air. It was a clear evening, with a beautiful sky full of stars helping the moon light our way.

I kept my distance, curling up on the bow of the boat, watching the stars and thinking. Looking at the stars reminded me of Mark and I camping out in the backyard. I wished he was with us. We were always safer together, and it meant that we at least had a witness.

I was hoping to spend most of the trip in that exact spot, and hopefully become invisible to the monster at the wheel. I was feeling peaceful and calm when a sudden splash beside the boat startled me. Then Pop called for me. Not knowing what the splash was, I wondered if we'd hit something.

My body was reacting to the feelings invoked by his voice. My mouth got dry suddenly, and it became difficult to swallow. I was hesitant to trust him but I knew I had to respond because even with Uncle Eddie on the boat, it was as if I was alone with Pop. I think what happened next was the reason he wanted me on this trip.

I walked cautiously down the side of the boat. My hand gripped the silver rail secured to the top of the cabin that ran from the bow to the stern of the boat. I was hanging onto the rail for dear life in case he decided to make a quick move and throw me overboard. I kept running all the past scenarios in my head, but couldn't figure out what was happening.

When I got down to the captain's level, I timidly said, "Yes, sir."

"Get up here and steer the boat. I need to check on the engine. Something sounds funny."

As usual, it wasn't a request but a command. I felt relieved, thinking maybe he wasn't going to bother me with Uncle Eddie on board.

I proudly climbed into the captain's chair and began steering the boat. He told me to leave the throttle alone and keep the course he had set. He said not to let the compass move off the large "E." I obeyed, thinking I was finally feeling his acceptance. I started to lower my guard and relax into my role of captain. I could feel the wind blowing on my face and smell the pure ocean air. All of the lights on the vessel were off except for the green and red navigation lights, the evening was simply beautiful.

He climbed down and lifted the doors of the engine room like they were made of paper. As the door was raised you could hear the roar of the engine get louder with every inch of the door being opened. Turning on his flash light, he stepped down onto the first rung of the ladder. He turned back and looked at me very confused, "I am having a hard time seeing anything." I turned to look at him and I could see that half of his body was down by one of the engines.

"Come down here and check the engine," he said. "I'm too big to get behind it." I was not sure I believed him because I saw him behind the engines before we left the docks. He knew I was terrified of the engine room especially at night.

Looking at him with huge eyes, "I am scared to do that, because it is so dark down there."

He looked cold and mean as he held out his hand to me. "I know you're scared," he said. "But I need you to do this for me." Going back to my original philosophy that he would not do anything to me while Uncle Eddie is here I thought that I might be safe to do this but I was still concerned.

I tried to think of a way to get out of it, but there didn't seem to be any alternative. He caught me off guard and I felt defenseless.

Suddenly he yelled, "Get your fucking ass down here now!" Realizing quickly that my options were limited I had to react.

"I'm steering the boat. If I leave, it could go off course," I said. This sounded logical to me and I was praying that he would go for it. With a demon like voice he retaliated, "You idiot," he said loudly. "I dropped the anchor, and you've been steering the damn boat in neutral."

I frantically started looking around. I couldn't tell we were not moving because I had no landmarks to which I could compare our positioning. There was nothing but water to see in every direction. I had no idea. I thought we were just moving slowly because he wanted to go in the engine room. I didn't notice there was no wake because the waves kept hitting the side of the boat. I was panicking now, desperate to find somewhere to go, and knowing there was no other place.

He yelled at me again and said, "Don't make me come up there and get you. Get down here now."

I saw no other way so I moved, but very slowly, making as much noise as possible, screaming as loudly as I could, "Okay, I'm on my way down."

Still trying to come up with some type of alternative I continued screaming, "Don't you think Uncle Eddie would be better help than me," determined to wake him out of a drunken sleep.

He said, "Nice try, but Eddie is so drunk he won't wake up if we're sinking." Realizing he was more correct than not, I continued to move towards the engine door. The closer I got the worse the smell of exhaust and oil became. Finally reaching the edge of the door opening unable to hear because of roar of the engine I became a zombie and could feel myself becoming disconnected from my body, preparing for the worst.

I stood in front of him as he sat on the deck, with his feet dangling, and we were eye to eye. "Just climb down there and check the spot where I have the flashlight pointed," he said. Knowing I couldn't trust him I was afraid I would get down there and wouldn't be able to see anything. I responded emotionlessly.

"I need a light to be able to see." He put his hand on my shoulder and started pushing me back towards the engine. I was trembling all over convinced he was going to try and shove me down into the engines without using the ladder.

"Just go on down. I'll shine till you get in the right spot, then I'll hand it to you," he said.

Again left with no choice, I moved closer to the little area of light.

Suddenly he stopped me with his beefy hand. "Before you go down there, take off your shorts and shirt so you won't get anything on them."

His games were starting and this particular one was getting ridiculous. "I'll tuck my shirt into my shorts, and it'll be fine." I looped my arm around one of the ladder steps and started tucking in my shirt. He stopped me in mid movement and grabbed my wrist. "That won't be good enough. Strip to your underwear and get in that engine room. I'm not going to risk your clothes getting caught in the engine," he said brusquely.

His logic made no sense to me, but I was more afraid of being thrown overboard. Realizing that I was standing on a ladder with heat blowing up on me from the engines, the smell of exhaust pillaging the air I was breathing, the sound of the engine absorbing every word I spoke I was stuck so I cautiously took off my shorts and shirt.

As I again started down, I looked around to see that the door hadn't been secured. He was holding it and I just wanted to get it over with so I continued my descent. "Could you please shine the light so I can see where I am stepping?" He leaned down so the light would go in further. I could feel sweat start to bead up on my forehead and I saw water with an oily residue on it gently splashing against the sides of the boat. I felt that I was making my way down into hell.

The engine was protected from the water because it was built on a raised platform and at eye level to make working on it easier. As I got to the bottom rung of the ladder, I was trying to find a place to put my foot so I could stand. I saw two boards that were side by side and determined they would be the best place to step first.

As my foot touched the first board, I felt the oil and gas tainted water gently lap over it. I could no longer hear anything at all from the deck above because of the roar of the engines. Cringing from the feeling of the water and not knowing what could be lurking in the darkness around me I screamed as loudly as I could up to the deck. I didn't know if the water was normal nor did I know how deep it was. "Is it normal for water to be in the bottom of the boat like this?" I could barely make out what he had said but didn't see him react too harshly so I assumed it was okay.

Once my footing was secured, I looked back at him and said, "Now shine the light on the area you need me to look at." Briefly the light from above disappeared and then suddenly the engines turned off. I reached out for the ladder trying to feel my way around scared of what I was touching but more frightened to be down in this dark hole with no light. "Please bring back the light, I can't see and I am really freaking out!"

Suddenly I could see the light shaking above on the deck and getting brighter with every step he took towards the opening. I had both of my hands on the ladder and one foot. He came back to the edge and shined the light directly in my eyes. The brightness of the light and the darkness I was just exposed to blinded me. "I can't see when you are shining the light right in my face like that. Will you shine the light on what it is you need for me to look at behind the engine so I can get out of here?" My voice was screechy and breaking as I stepped back off of the ladder to shield my eyes.

"Okay," he said solemnly. "But first, I need to know that you will do everything I ask you to do." Thinking he was talking about the engine, but based on his tone, I could not tell. I thought it was an odd demand so I didn't say okay immediately. I wanted further clarification of what he meant.

"Why?" I asked insistently trying to look around the light that was shining in my eyes.

He moved the heavy door and acted as if he were going to lower the door and close me down there and said again, "I need to know that you will do *everything* I ask you to do while you are on this trip with me."

Confused, I said, "It really depends on what you mean by everything. I'll do what I can, but I don't know if I can do everything." I had never seen him like this before but I knew that I could not agree to something I could not complete because the consequences could be too great.

He said, "That's not good enough." And he dropped the door, leaving me in total darkness.

I could feel the water on my feet, barely able to breath because of the horrible odor. It went from being so loud to deafeningly quiet. All I could hear was him pacing loudly on the door above my head and the water sloshing. The water splashed against the sides of the boat, and continued to lap across my feet. The constant submersion of them in water, gas and oil was starting to act like a meat tenderizer and cause them to burn. I held my hands out to try and find the ladder to crawl back onto so I could get my feet out of the water but I had become disoriented. I had my hands out and I thought I was in the right area and then I felt the singe of the engines against my hands.

I was startled and didn't want to move my feet from the board that they were on and started to sway back and forth. It was inevitable, I lost my balance and the left side of my body fell against the engine and it felt like someone was pouring scalding water against my side. I could smell my flesh burning, but I still couldn't see anything in front of me. I fell down into the disgusting water, I could feel the oil and gas seep in through my newly opened burn wounds. This place was the darkest place I had ever been and all I wanted to do was get out.

He yelled through the door, "I need to hear you say you will do *everything* I ask you to do while you are here."

Even as frightened as I was, I still said, "It will depend on what you want me to do. What if you ask me to do something I don't know how to do?"

I knew being in this darkness was horrible but committing to something that I was not sure of with him could be even worse.

When I got no response, I began to panic again and started screaming as loud as I could. I finally found the ladder and pulled myself up out of the water. As I put my foot on the bottom rung of the ladder and pull myself out of the water I could feel my underwear drenched and burning my genitals and anus. I climbed up to the top of the ladder and started pushing on the door as hard as I could. I could feel the door open slightly and as the door started to lift I could see the moonlight start to shine through the crack.

I used all of my body to try and push the door all the way open when all of the sudden I heard the sound of someone running and then a sudden thud that shut the door onto my head. He had run from the captain's chair across the deck to stomp onto the door to keep me from getting out. I fell off of the ladder and back into the water below. My back had hit the boards that I was originally standing on and I froze briefly wondering if anything was broken. I got back up and stood on top of the boards to keep as much of my body out of the water as possible. My feet were burning so badly that I could barely stand. All the noise finally woke Uncle Eddie.

"Eddie, get your drunk ass back in bed," I could hear Pop say. I started screaming at the top of my lungs

"Uncle Eddie please help me, please! I am down here by the engines, please help me!" I paused and heard nothing.

Uncle Eddie ignored my cries or couldn't figure out where I was and said, "Son," the name all of his friends and family called him, "you can't do this to that boy." I was shocked. He knew exactly what was going on and he would not help me out of here.

Pop said, "Who's going to stop me? Just go back to bed."

I lowered myself down to sit on the boards my feet were standing on and wrapped my arms around my knees.

I guess I wasn't the only one afraid of Pop. My heart sank as Uncle Eddie crossed the deck and walked back down the stairs to the cabin, slamming the door.

I couldn't believe it. *Why was Pop doing this to me? What was going on up there? What had I done to make Pop so mad?*

I searched my imagination for ways to calm myself. It seemed to help if I closed my eyes, but the smell was so strong, it made me nauseous. When I heard Pop walking away, I truly began to panic.

I yelled, "Wait. Wait. Please don't leave me down here." I knew that by this time I had already been down there for at least an hour. The engines had started to cool off and it went from being boiling hot to freezing.

He stopped and said, "All you have to do is everything I ask."

I hesitated and finally asked, "What are you going to ask me to do?"

"I have to hear that you agree to do everything, or else I'll just leave you down there with the engine."

He gave me a horrible choice once again, but I found myself thinking it might be better to stand in the dark than be stuck up there with him. I truly thought I was going to die, alone and cold in the dark, just because I wouldn't let him do what he wanted.

The quiet was broken by the engine starting. I felt the intense heat build back up from the engines, and the exhaust fumes became unbearable. I was screaming and crying. I'd never been so frightened. He left the engine running for about five minutes, and then turned it off and raised the door above me. I was gasping for air, and I was certain he was going to kill me. I refused to look up at him and I stayed in my position with my arms around my legs.

He looked at me and said, "So, will you do *everything* I ask you to do?"

Wanting to say no but knowing that death was certain if I stayed down there with the carbon dioxide I realized I was totally defeated and said, "Fine. I'll do everything you want me to do."

I decided I had a better chance of surviving on deck.

He reached in to give me a hand up, but I bypassed it and took the ladder instead.

I quickly moved to the ladder and placed both hands on each side. When my foot first made contact with the step I could feel the pain shoot all the way through my body. It felt like someone was forcing me to walk on hot metal rods. With each step it became more and more difficult. I started using my hands to pull myself up just to alleviate some of the pressure on my feet. "You're one hard-headed boy, do you know that?" he said as if I had conquered one of his manhood tests.

I ignored his words and looked down at my feet. I just knew they were going to rot off. They were hurting badly. I could hardly walk, and they were wrinkled from being submerged for so long. When I got to the top step, I literally fell onto the floor and drew in big gulps of the fresh air, which led to a coughing fit. I saw the burn marks on my left side from where I had fallen onto the engine. The wounds were oozing and bloody. I continued to do an assessment and realized that when I fell on my back I had cut my leg and arm when I had landed, I was bruising already and reeked.

He told me to take off my underwear and without any argument, I reached down to the disgusting remnants of my underwear and I pulled them down to my knees and pulled my knees to my chest. I wanted to take them all the way off but not in front of him, I wanted to go and shower and throw them away.

"Take them all the way off," he said, his voice heavy and course.

Afraid to challenge him and exhausted I slid them down to my feet and laid them on the deck beside me. He leaned down and kissed my cheek, saying, "You smell like gas fumes and piss." Helping me up, he added, "Jump in the water and get yourself washed off."

I looked at him in astonishment. *We're in the ocean at night, and he wants me to jump in the water? Oh my God this is it, he is going to drown me and tell my mother I jumped over board and they couldn't find me.*

Thinking quickly, I asked, "Why can't I just shower in the cabin?" The pain was starting to subside because my adrenaline was kicking in. My heart was beating a million miles a minute.

"I don't want you waking Eddie up. Jump in the water." I didn't want to challenge him and I had resolved to the fact that I was getting ready to die. I closed my eyes and started to pray, thanking God for Charlie and Nelly. He reached down and snatched me up by my arm.

"Come on," he urged. "I won't leave you, and nothing will get you."

That didn't sound too reassuring, but all I wanted to do was survive and get back home and hopefully never see him again.

He pulled me up off of the deck and I covered my penis with my hands.

He pushed me to the back of the boat where another ladder extends down so you can slowly submerge yourself in the water. My foot touched the top step and pain shot through my calf, when my second foot touched; I felt the same pain in the other calf. As I got closer to the water, my heart beat faster and faster.

I had never been in the ocean at night. I lowered myself into the water, and the salt began stinging my burns and cuts. All I could do was push away the pain and think about all the things I would do when I got home.

I kept my hold on the ladder with one hand and splashed water over my face and body with the other, trying to get myself clean. The ocean water was slicing through my burns and cuts like alcohol in an open wound. I could taste the salt from the water in my mouth and for it to be night time it was so much brighter than I thought it would be.

Abruptly I heard another command, "Get back up here now."

As I reached the top rung, I saw he was completely naked and had an erection. *He put me through all of that and now he wants me to have sex with him? What a freak.*

I briefly considered jumping back into the water and drowning myself, but I didn't want people to think my death was a simple suicide. Besides, if I did that, I wouldn't be anyone's angel, and I'd never see Mark again because suicide was a sin.

I got to the top and sat on the edge of the boat, just looking at him warily.

He said, "Come over here and get on your knees." Wishing Uncle Eddie would come back outside to try and talk him out of it. I remained where I was; not wanting to do what he had asked.

"Your only other option is to go back to the engine room," he said evenly.

My other option is to die, but I didn't want this as an alternative.

In reality, I had no choice, so I crawled over to him on my knees unable to put any pressure on my feet and he forced me to perform oral sex on him. With every thrust I gagged and eventually puked all over his groin, but he just shoved my face into it and kept going.

I was being smothered by my vomit all over his clammy flesh and the odor was horrible. He kept pushing, and I could taste the stomach acid in my throw up. He finally finished and made me put my clothes on and go down into the cabin.

As I walked down the steps wiping my stomach contents off of my face, Uncle Eddie looked at me and drunkenly asked, "You all right?" I stared at him incredulity. He was awake the entire time and knew exactly what was going on. I was not sure who was sicker, Pop for doing it or Uncle Eddie doing nothing to help me.

I mumbled, "Yeah," just to avoid talking to the drunk and walked around him.

I went to the bathroom and brushed my teeth and cleaned myself up. When I came out, I was completely dressed, and I climbed up into the smallest area of the cabin at the bow of the boat, where I felt most secure. There was only one way in and one way out of this area, so if he came for me during the night I knew I'd be able to see him coming.

When I was about six years old, Mamma O had beautiful red velvet bedspreads made for the twin beds she had given to me. They were so soft to the touch, almost like rubbing the soft belly of a puppy. I would lie in my bed at night finally feeling safe and secure with the weight of the red velvet covers pressing and hugging my body tightly. I always fantasized that the weight of the covers were actually Nelly holding her arms around me as tightly as she could while I would drift off to sleep. I fantasized about having these covers with me as I dozed off to sleep in the bow of the boat.

Uncle Eddie was the first one up the next morning, and he had coffee and breakfast ready. I stepped out of my sleeping area and cautiously looked around. Pop was still sleeping so I slowly placed my feet on the ground. Flashbacks started to come to me quickly of last night's events unfortunately realizing it was not a nightmare.

I looked down at my feet and they were pink, black and brown from the chemicals and water. They were hurting worse than the night before. I slowly moved my hand up to feel my side and the newly formed scabs that were covering the sores from where I had been burned. They were tacky to the touch and not doing a good job of covering the horrific events that had taken place. I walked, as best as I could, past Pop trying not to wake him. One foot at a time, I stepped out of the cabin.

I looked at Uncle Eddie, and he toasted me with a beer, saying, "To the hair of the dog that bit me."

I didn't know what he meant. I thought he meant it was the same beer that got him drunk last night. I could tell he was feeling remorseful for his lack of actions from the night before.

I had nothing to say to him so I grabbed some breakfast and again took up my position on the bow of the boat and was transfixed by the sound of nothing but the ocean and the air. I was day dreaming about being home and seeing Nelly and spending the afternoons riding Charlie.

During my day dream I became concerned, realizing I had only made it through one night of this trip with one more to go. My wonderful peace was broken only by the fear of what he would ask me to do next. I tried to think of things I could do to keep it from happening. *Maybe I could get Uncle Eddie to do something other than drink beer.*

Trying to plan ahead before Pop waked up, I went back to the deck of the boat and asked Uncle Eddie if he would like to play a game or something with me later on. He said, "Sure, if it can be a drinking game." Well, there went that idea. I hated the smell and taste of beer and the last thing I wanted to do was put me in a place where I could not be in control. I went back to the bow of the boat when I heard Pop moving around below. During the day I would sneak down into the cabin to use the rest room and grab food to eat without either of them knowing by dropping down from the top of the boat through the window in my sleeping area.

My paranoia and concern grew as the day stretched on. Uncle Eddie was drunk again by the time lunch rolled around, he was swaying more than the boat was. He was trying to fix himself a lunch but gave up and passed out on the deck.

I hoped I would be out of harm's way as long as it was daylight and Uncle Eddie on the deck. I thought surely Pop wouldn't try anything right in front of Eddie.

Clouds rolled in, and I noticed there weren't as many boats around us. I wondered if we'd wandered off course. I'd never been out on the ocean that far. It was beautiful but boring, and I mostly just wanted to get back home.

I was lying on the bow reading my book when I again heard a loud splash in the water. This time I knew what it was. He'd dropped the anchor again.

I panicked. *How does he know how deep the water is and that we are not just drifting around out here?* Then I remembered him telling my uncle about the new depth-measuring tool he bought so he wouldn't run the risk of hitting a sand bar. I knew now he hadn't bought it because he feared sand bars.

He bought it to know when he could drop his anchor overboard and abuse me.

When I heard him call my name, I pretended I didn't hear anything. I was hoping he'd yell loud enough to wake up Uncle Eddie. He called again and again; I just ignored him. I waited for a few minutes and didn't hear anything else, so I thought that he gave up.

All of the sudden the hatch door on the bow of the boat that leads down into the cabin where I was sleeping opened. I saw the door slowly rise and I knew it was him. I badly wanted to stomp on it as he had done to me with the door of the engine. If I did this though, I would have even more hell to pay for the rest of the trip back. He popped his head out. "Didn't you hear me calling you?" Trying to play dumb and think of reasons why I couldn't have heard him I responded, "Um . . . no, I couldn't hear because of the wind."

Not really phased by my response or truly looking for one he tapped me on my leg and said, "I need you to come down here and help me with something."

"What do you need help with?" I was not going to get myself into a situation like I was in last night. I refused to be locked back in that dark room. I was hurting all over and having a hard time walking as it was and I was at the point where I would jump on Uncle Eddie if I had to just to get him to wake up.

"Stop asking so many questions and get down here," he said roughly.

I reluctantly got up and walked to the cabin door. As I passed, I nonchalantly pushed Uncle Eddie out of his chair to wake him up. I stopped in my tracks when a menacing voice said, "Unless you want to wind up in the same situation you were in yesterday, you'll get into this hatch now."

I immediately headed for the circular opening in the bow of the boat, dropping my book first, hoping it might hit him on the head. No such luck. It missed, and I slowly began to lower myself into the hatch and accidentally hit my burn on the way down. The pain reminded me of my horrible time last night and made me truly fear what was in store for me now.

When I got into the cabin, he was naked and waiting. Once again, I got sick to my stomach not knowing what to do. As soon as I was inside, he turned to lock the cabin door. While his back was to me I darted back toward the hatch door but I could not move as fast as normal because of the previous night's events. I was immediately grabbed by the back of my hair and thrown down onto the dining table in the kitchenette area. He had lowered it to the same height as the benches, and he had moved the fishing poles that were there before behind the bench. Fear and terror rushed over me, afraid that he would do to me again something that was tormenting and painful.

I looked at him as if he were fully dressed and said, "What do you need?"

His fierce eyes raked over me and he angrily said, "I need you to get naked and sit on this table." I was not going to have something happen to me again without a fight.

"Why?" I asked, knowing it would only infuriate him. At this point I didn't care. I thought I had my get-away plotted. I was going to run past him, unlock the door, burst out onto the deck and wake up Uncle Eddie. It would be difficult for him to explain running after me naked.

As he raised his hand to hit me in the head I saw my opportunity and took it. I ducked from his fist and bolted for the door. I think I must have jumped from the floor to the top step like a cat. I didn't feel any pain at all only adrenaline rushing through my veins.

I never looked back to see where he was all I wanted to do once again was get out of this prison. I was sick of him and just wanted it all to end. As I reached for the door knob, I felt a hand grab my hair again. I quickly peered out of the crack in the door while at the top step. I could see Uncle Eddie through the crack. He was awake and walking around.

This was it, he will hear me and come running in to keep anything from happening.

I made exaggerated moves to knock over anything at all to get Uncle Eddie's attention. While he was dragging me across the floor I could feel the carpet burning my back. I was knocking over dishes that were on the counter, kicking the cabinets and screaming at the top of my lungs. I knew that the engines were loud but I didn't think they would be too loud to hear me begging for him not to hurt me again. He didn't appear to hear anything.

I continued to scream until Pop covered my mouth with his hand. I could smell the horrific odor of his skin up against my nose. It smelled like he had been filleting dead fish and had never once washed his hands. I knew there was no way Uncle Eddie couldn't have heard me. I was fighting and hitting Pop in the face, and then he gave me a solid blow to my stomach that knocked the breath out of me. I stopped instantly and he moved his hand.

Trying to catch my breath, he picked me up like I was nothing more than a rag doll and threw me onto the table, which was waist high for him. He yanked me on my side and began pulling off my shorts. I was trying to breathe and continued to fight him.

He grabbed my hands and put them behind my back and I started to feel him slip something around them. My eyes got huge because I realized he was tying them together with fishing line. I started to plead, "Please don't, oh my God, please don't do this to me Pop, please!" With my hands tied, there was nothing more I could do and I just started staring at the ceiling.

I had no more fight left in me. I just lay there like I was a corpse. He tore my shorts off and pulled me to the edge of the table and flipped me on my back. My genitals and anus were still raw from the oil and gas chemicals I was exposed to down by the engines. Without any lubricant once again, he shoved himself inside me and I could feel my skin rip apart while his drips of sweat fell onto my face and body. With every thrust I could feel my skin rip more and I was so detached I couldn't feel anything.

While my head was banging up against the wall of the cabin I looked over at the door, I saw Uncle Eddie outside the cabin window. I kept thinking he'd hear me screaming and crying so I started screaming louder. I was praying he'd do something.

My screams became so loud that Pop shoved his fingers in my mouth. He placed them so far down I couldn't breathe and I was gagging. I bit down on them, and the harder I tried to bite, the more he would close his hand and it felt like he was going to pull my lower jaw off of my skull. I tried moving around to try and get him out of me. The more I moved the more I could feel the fishing line cutting into my wrist. I finally just put my head back and felt myself leave my body.

The ethereal feeling of knowing that your physical body is present but that mentally you have completely disconnected from your body is not a feeling you should experience at age thirteen. I believed this monster was not human at all, simply because of his mindless and soulless ability to attack vulnerable children and encourage them to do what he wanted out of fear. The entire time he was raping me I was completely unaware of what was happening to my body. It was as if I could see what was going on, but it was so unreal I could not stop it.

There was a knock on the cabin door, and Uncle Eddie said, "I need to use the bathroom." This brought me back and I could feel him still inside me, slamming himself into me so hard that it felt like my intestines were going to be ripped out.

"Piss off the side of the boat," Pop said. "I'm busy" he said with heaving breathing, like he was running a marathon. Uncle Eddie was truly trying to help me this time. I tried to raise my body up and he shoved me back down onto the table and threw his gross sweaty body against me to keep me pinned down.

"I need to take a shit. Besides, what are you doing in there?" Uncle Eddie said. I tried to scream and again, he shoved his hand in my mouth. Finally I couldn't take it anymore and tears started rolling out of my eyes.

"I'm bonding with my grandson. Just go away," was Pop's angry reply. I knew there was nothing more I or anyone else could do until he was done.

"Son, you can't continue to do this," Eddie said sternly.

"Oh, yeah, Eddie, what are you going to do about it? You and I used to do this all the time."

You and I used to do this all of the time. With those words, my heart just broke. All along, Uncle Eddie knew what was happening, and all along, I had been hoping he would save me. In actuality, he probably wanted to do the same thing to me.

With his final thrust, Pop finally finished. There was blood all over the kitchen table, my legs, the floor and my crotch.

He reached down taking a deep breath and said, "Wow, you really wore me out that time."

I didn't move or say a word. I just looked up at the ceiling. My hands still bound behind me. I could feel myself slide around on the table in my own blood when I tried to sit up.

"Would you please untie my hands? I can't feel my fingers." I said quietly.

"Sure let me finish getting dressed."

I sat there bleeding with the fishing line cutting into my wrists and my head hanging low between my shoulders. Finally he came over with his fishing knife and cut the line. I could feel the blood rush to my finger tips and when I moved my arms back in front and I could feel the stiffness from them being in the same position for so long.

I looked down at my hands and wrists and couldn't tell where the cuts actually were because there was so much blood. I reached down and slowly pulled my shorts up over my bloody legs and I could feel his semen that he got all over my shorts stick to body.

He stopped me and said, "Go jump into the ocean again to clean yourself off."

Why does he want me to do this all of the time. Why can't I just take a shower?

"I'd rather have a shower."

He said, "Your uncle Eddie needs to take a shit, and that comes before you."

How poetic. I wasn't even worth more than a shit.

"That's fine, I will just wait for him and then I will shower after that."

I didn't want to get into the salty ocean because I was afraid that the water would hurt my open wounds too much.

When I told Pop that, he walked over to me, pulled my clothes off, picked me up naked and carried me to the deck. As I came up the steps, hanging naked over Pops shoulder bloody and bruised, I looked at the expression on Uncle Eddies face.

He seemed surprised to see the blood on my hands and coming from my ass, and he said, "Son, what have you done?"

Still in shock over what had taken place it still did not register with me the extent of what had happened.

He continued across the boat deck to the back of the boat. I was hanging over his shoulder like a sand bag and without warning he picked me up over his head and tossed me overboard.

I had no idea what was happening. I was falling but I didn't know what was below me. I tried to turn my body around to make sure I was not going to land on the ladder behind the boat. I was scared because of the blood I had all over me might attract sharks.

Then suddenly, my mind stopped when my body hit the salt water, it felt like someone was slicing me with razor blades and pouring lemon juice all over me. My burns were stinging, the cuts on my wrists felt like they were on fire. My ass felt like someone was shoving a broken glass bottle up my rectum. All those cuts and burns made it feel like I was swimming in a vat of acid.

Frantically trying to get out of the water I went swimming back to the boat that was my torture chamber. I didn't know where else to go.

I climbed back up the ladder; Uncle Eddie was standing there with a towel. Again, he asked me if I was all right.

I looked at him and said, "How much longer is this trip going to last?"

"We should be docking in the morning," he said quietly.

"All I have to do is get through the night, and I'll be fine." *I know I can't count on you for shit.*

Fortunately that night the weather became pretty rough, so I went down into the cabin to my little secure cubby hole. I was bounced all over the place and didn't get much sleep, but it was still better than dealing with the old bastard on deck. Finally the waves subsided and, for a change, Uncle Eddie was somewhat sober and was steering the boat. I heard Pop come into the cabin to use the restroom. When he was finished, I heard the toilet flush and then I fell asleep.

The next morning when I awoke, Pop was in my sleeping quarters. I was so emotionally drained that when he forced me to perform oral sex, I did it without protest.

I was thankful to hear Uncle Eddie yell for Pop and say, "Hey, I see the marina."

When Pop was finished, he looked at me and said in a cold, hard voice, "If you tell anyone about this trip, I'll kill you."

I knew he was telling the truth.

The first person I saw when we docked that day was Mom. She came running up to me, all smiles, and said, "It's so wonderful to see you. I missed you."

"I missed you too," I said blandly. "Can we go home?"

She was still smiling as she said, "Sure. But you need to help your grandfather clean the boat." Having to go back to that boat and clean up the series of hell he put me through was the last thing I was interested in doing.

"I really think he can do that without me," and I continued walking towards the car.

Her voice became stern, "Young man, don't be so ungrateful for what your grandparents are doing for us. Now go over there and help him clean the boat."

I threw what I had into her car and went back to the boat.

"Pop, Mom wants me to help you clean up the boat. What do you want me to do?" I already knew what he had in mind for me to do. He wouldn't face what he had done to me and I had to clean up the torturous path he had left behind.

Truly emotionless, I went down into the cabin, where I wiped my dried blood off of the kitchenette table. I scrubbed my vomit off of the deck floor, picked up my stained and bloody old shirt and shorts. I put it in my bag, went to the bathroom and wiped the tears from my face, and felt myself shift to a new level of numbness toward my family.

When I'd done everything Pop told me to do, I went back to Mom, and she asked me if I'd told Pop good-bye. I turned around and said, "Good-bye, "without any sincerity He smiled, looking like he owned me, and said, "Don't worry. We'll have some fun again soon, and remember what I told you." *How could I ever forget? What you have done to me is unforgivable.*

I hurried to the car with her behind me telling me how rude I was just to walk away like that.

Once we got back home, I went immediately into the shower and once I had washed off that nightmare of a trip I went looking for Nelly. She was washing clothes and I went running up to her and she stopped me with her eyes huge.

"Honey, what did that monster do to you?" She immediately saw the cuts on my arms, wrists and legs. Mom never even noticed the bruises and cuts I had all over my body.

"Don't worry about it, I am here with you now and remember what doesn't kill me only makes me stronger. I am going to go see Charlie I just wanted you to know that I love you too."

She put her hand on my face and said, "You don't need to worry about anything because this is not in your hands now. What he has done, he will never be forgiven for."

Without even having to tell her a word about the trip, she was able to look into my eyes and know every single event that took place. She knew me better than any other person in the world.

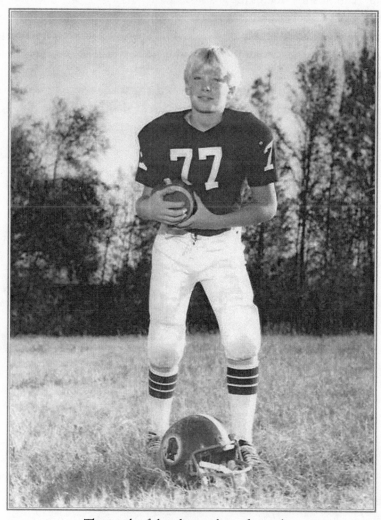

The result of the photo taken of me when
I was so sick, forcing myself to smile.

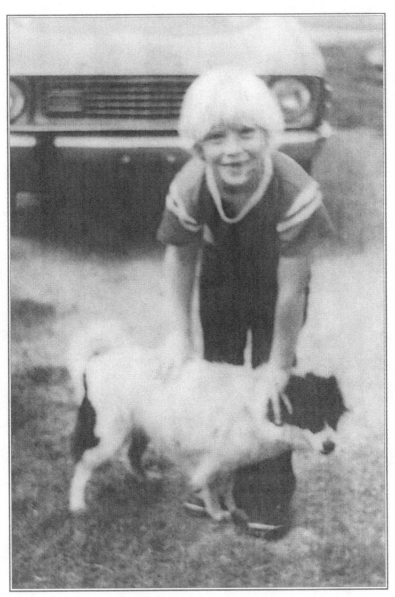

A picture of me and my Lucky.

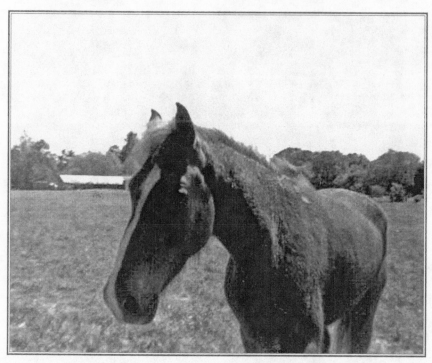

Charlie in the winter time when I first got him.

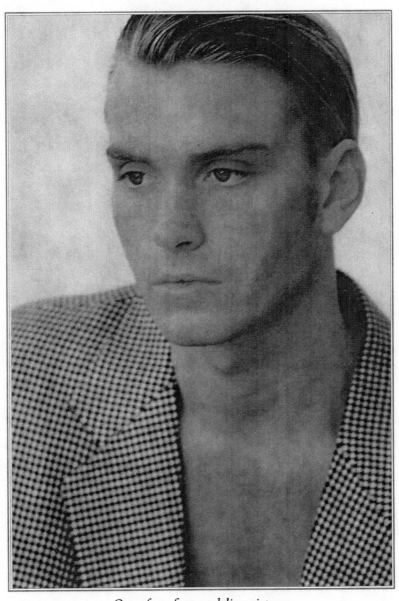

One of my first modeling pictures

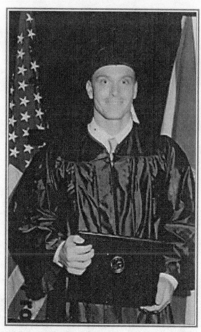

Me the moment I got off of the stage after receiving my college diploma.

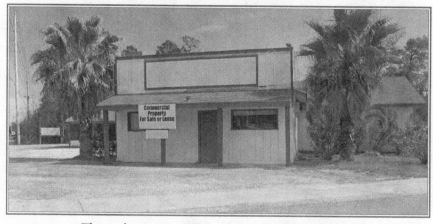

*This is the store, in 2010, where I sought refuge and
waited on my father to come and pick me up.*

CHAPTER 6

LESSONS FROM LOVE

With a final effort to feel normal again, I decided to pitch the idea to my mother that she and I move to Panama City to be closer to Aunt Patricia and Uncle Nick. I was sure we'd have some type of normalcy and peace by living close to them. Aunt Patricia was an amazing lady with the beauty of Ava Gardner and the singing voice of Judy Garland. She always made herself available to listen to any crazy idea or thought I might have had and never judged me. She was very supportive of my mother, and she was one of the few people I always felt safe around because of her unconditional love and her view on life. She had sacrificed her dreams to support my uncle with his career. She stayed busy coordinating his calendar, cooking all of the meals, and being a sounding board for the congregation he had built that held him in such high standards. Regardless of her schedule or day, she always made time for me.

Uncle Nick was a Methodist preacher and was not around very often because his congregation kept him busy during the week and of course on Sundays. When he was around, he was always complaining or barking orders to the people around him. I always found it ironic that a man of God had no patience or appreciation for the people in his life.

I heard Mom's car pull into the driveway, which sobered me from my thoughts of living in Panama City. I immediately got butterflies in my stomach.

How should I start this of? Should I meet her at the door or should I wait for her to come in and sit down?

The front door opened and immediately as the door closed Mom yelled "I'm home."

I took a deep breath and just thought, *what would Nelly tell me to do? I could hear her voice telling me, "there is nothing for you to worry about... trust yourself...what is the worst thing she could say to you?" The worst thing could be that she would tell me I am being selfish and that she wants to stay here for the rest of her life. Either way I am willing to take the chance because if that is the worst thing that she could say it will get me ready for my future.*

With her words in my head I just went for it, "Hey Mom, how was your day today?"

"It was long and I am tired, how was yours?" She always sounded so defeated with her tone when she had gotten off work as if she had just worked twenty hours. Instead of doing anything constructive to make her day better she would just sit in her chair and turn on the television to become transfixed on something other than her life.

Knowing I really had to up my enthusiasm to spark her interest, I really had to over exaggerate my tone to get her attention. I had to balance it without sounding sarcastic but something more of a huge discovery.

"It was great and I came up with an incredible idea that I think makes a lot of sense and you will really like it but I need for you to listen to all of it before you say anything"

Okay, you can't back out of this now, be careful but convincing and hope that you sound enthusiastic enough.

She slowly turned her head and looked at me and I knew I had pitched the start of the idea well. I didn't want to lose her interest so I continued.

"You know how great Aunt Patricia and Uncle Nick are and how wonderful they are to us," I said with convincing enthusiasm.

"Yes." With her response, she slowly put down the remote on the table beside her chair, and I knew I had hit on something interesting to her.

"Well, I was thinking it would be great if we could all live in the same town, because you hate living here in Selma and I can't stand it either, Evelyn is moving away to live with Dad and I just think it would be a great time for us to make a new start."

She paused for a moment, as if actually to think about what I was saying.

I couldn't believe it she was really contemplating it as an option, and I started to ramble quickly as if to finish my sale.

"You know that they love us, and I am sure they will help us get settled and pick a good area for us to live that would be in a good school district," and with those words of excitement came the words that were all-encompassing and to the point.

Her face went from a fantasy glow to anger and frustration and her tone changed as if to say I was not being realistic and then her words loudly hit the air.

"No, no, no."

With my hope suddenly shifting to despair, I managed to squeak out, "but why not?"

"I don't have enough money to move us to Florida." She said as if I were chastising her.

She thought I understood that, but what she didn't understand was my soul was being strangled a little bit every day staying in Selma.

I continued with my argument trying to convince her everything would be alright and help eliminate her financial concerns.

"The three of us would be fine living in Florida; I just know we will be. Between Dad's child support and moving into a smaller house and into a city that has better jobs I know it will be better."

She looked at me with a very perplexed look and asked, "What do you mean the three of us?"

"You, Charlie, and me," I replied.

"Of course, Charlie," her tone changed as if the reality of us moving was just a fantasy. She grabbed her cigarette case and as she pulled out a cigarette she proceeded with her final argument. "Well, son, if you bring Charlie along, then we'll need even more money. Horses are very expensive."

I was not going to give up and all I wanted her to do was listen to me and hear the possibilities and not be so bogged down in the impossibilities.

"Please put down your cigarette and listen to me. Dad will pay for Charlie," I commented with conviction.

She looked at me, rolled her eyes and put the cigarette she had been struggling to get out of her cigarette case between her lips. Not even looking at me she flippantly dismissed the thought.

"Your dad won't even pay for your education, much less pay your horse's bills,"

"Mom, I don't care. We can work it out. Can't we just move?" I pleaded.

Lighting her cigarette with a large inhale she paused and then said as she released the toxic smoke,

"We can't afford it, and that's final," and she picked up the remote and turned on the television to tune me out.

Defeated, I slowly walked back to my bedroom trying to not show my anger and frustration. Pulling from other conversations I had with Nelly I thought, *what can I do to make her realize how important this it to me? Nelly once told me that to love things don't focus so hard on holding on to them forever but instead keep them in your heart forever.*

For the first time I could feel what she was talking about. I knew what I had to do. It was the one thing I'd vowed never to do. If Mom knew this was something I am willing to do then she would understand how very important this move is to me.

I knew I had to do it to save myself. I also knew Charlie would want to help me if he could. I never doubted Charlie's love.

Eventually I got up the nerve to call Mr. Cochran, the man who had sold Charlie to us. He'd always said that if anything happened, he'd buy Charlie back. As I went to dial the last digit of his number, I hesitated. *What if I sell him and she still refuses to move. I will be stuck in this horrible place without Charlie and I couldn't stand the thought of that. When I talk to Mr. Cochran, maybe he will understand and he will have some advice or maybe he will refuse to buy Charlie back and he will tell Mom of my attempt.*

I dialed the last digit and the phone started to ring I frantically rationalized, *Maybe he is not home and if he doesn't answer, I'll call him back later.* I thought while leaning against the kitchen counter.

Then the second ring was interrupted "hello"

"Mr. Cochran?" I said with a cautious manner.

"Yes" inquisitively he responded.

"Hi, I am not sure if you remember me or not but I am the kid who bought Charlie from you"

"Of course I remember you. I think about Charlie almost every day and wonder how you two are doing."

I am glad that he remembers me but I wish he hated me for calling him. I hope he knows I am not a bad person for what I am about to ask.

"When we bought him you had mentioned that if there was ever a need for us to sell him you would be willing to buy him back. Is that still true?"

I closed my eyes, *please say no, please, say no,* I started chanting with my thoughts. Then negotiating the outcome, I considered, *if he says yes then it was meant to be?*

"Without a doubt that is true, why do you need to sell him? I thought you loved him?"

Immediately my heart sank. The idea was becoming a reality and I didn't want anyone to think that I did not love Charlie. My love for Charlie changed my life. He taught me humor because he unintentionally did the silliest things like stop mid-stride when a bird flew near him. You could see the paranoid look in his eyes, afraid that the bird would try and swoop down and carry him away. He weighed a ton but the smallest bird would scare him to paralysis. He would see a garbage can on the side of the street and walk cautiously past. He would widen his stance and drop down as if he were a small cat on the prowl trying to avoid being noticed. He also taught me how to love.

Knowing he was so dependent on me for certain things like eating and attention made me realize how important it was to be tender and attentive, even when the thing you are caring for is four times your size. He was a big baby and jovial as well. He would sneak up on me when I would clean out his stall and take his snout and hit me in my butt to try and push me out of his stall.

He taught me how to feel so the thought of someone thinking I didn't love him was almost enough for me to hang up the phone and just forget this as an option. I knew I had to do the right thing for both of us.

Detaching myself from the intense feelings I had for Charlie and looking at this more of a transaction instead of selling the only thing I have ever loved is what I had to do.

"I love him more than you could ever imagine which is why I needed to call you and ask you if you would buy him back"

Trying to keep my composure and not become an emotional wreck. I continued on and explained the situation and the reason why I needed to sell him. He was patient and sympathetic throughout the entire conversation.

"Mr. Cochran, I do need to ask you one thing. If I sell Charlie back to you and we don't move, I am not sure what I would do without him."

He interrupted me, "I tell you what, if you don't move you can come out here every day if you want and still treat Charlie as if he were your own, how does that sound?"

"That sounds incredible and I can't thank you enough."

"When would you like for me to come and get him from you?"

I had not thought this far ahead and really didn't have an answer. *I want to spend as much time with him as I can before he is no longer mine but I could also spend that time with him at Mr. Cochran's house based on his previous invite.*

"Mr. Cochran, are you sure I can come and see him anytime I want?"

"Absolutely"

I closed my eyes, and when I did I could feel the tears I had been holding back start to fall and I softly whispered "thank you God."

"Okay, will tomorrow work for you?" I said timidly.

"I will be there tomorrow around four o'clock."

That seemed so early to me but the reality is if he had told me in two years he would be there that would be too soon also.

"I will see you then"

"Before you hang up, does your mother know you are doing this?"

I knew if she found out she would try and keep it from happening because it was her only excuse at this point. I would eliminate her concern about Charlie being too expensive and also have money to move us down to Florida.

"No Sir, she does not and I would prefer that we keep it that way if you don't mind"

"I understand and I will see you tomorrow."

I hung up the phone and with confused feelings I fell to pieces. It was as if someone was tearing at my heart. I was so upset that I couldn't inhale due to the fact that so much of my body's energy was being used on my tears. I doubled over curling up into a ball and pulled my knees into my chest all in one movement. I felt like I couldn't continue. Both the emotional pain of selling Charlie and the physical strain of my body convulsing and hyperventilating from the agonizing heart break were almost too much to accept.

I didn't want to sell Charlie but at the same time I didn't want to keep going through the hell of living in Selma any longer.

I knew the most difficult step I needed to take was next, going to the barn to say good-bye to him.

Regaining my composure, I walked up toward the pasture. He must have seen me because he headed for the fence where I was. I paused, staring at him in disbelief, so thankful that this beautiful animal was mine. The pasture was lush and green which created the perfect background to pronounce his beautiful chestnut coat. He had the most wonderful swaggering walk, and as he got closer I could smell his incredible scent. He smelled like cut grass and sweet molasses from his feed. He always seemed to have a smile on his face as if to say, "Hey, don't worry about anything, you are with me now."

I broke down and thought I would never catch my breath knowing that the feeling of peace that I treasured so much was coming to an end. As he got closer, I threw my arms around his huge muscular neck, collapsing into his body holding on and never wanting to let go.

"Charlie, please know it was nothing that you have done and I hope you know how much I love you. I pray you understand or at least I want to believe that you do. You have been the best friend I have always wanted, and Mr. Cochran said I can come and see you anytime I want. I would give anything in this world if you could go with me. Please know you have been perfect and none of this is your fault."

I know he didn't understand a word I said, but his face looked like he could feel my pain. I stayed at the barn most of the evening, hoping that from our unspoken words he knew how much I loved him. When I finally got home, I went to bed, but was up again at four o'clock the next morning.

In twelve hours Charlie will be going back to his original home.

I put the pillow back over my head and tried to fall back asleep. I was struggling because I couldn't stop the images of the wonderful experiences Charlie had brought to my life. Riding down to the edge of the river, tying him up loosely to a tree and me going swimming and talking and laughing at him for hours while I frolicked around in the water. The experience of riding him bareback and really connecting with something for the first time was the greatest reward. I always knew I was safe with him and that he would be there to protect me. Finally I drifted off to sleep.

That afternoon, as we had agreed, Mr. Cochran arrived with his horse trailer in tow. He backed down the long entry way to the barn and I came walking up to the side of his truck. He jumped out with a smile on his face that quickly turned to concern when he saw how red and swollen my eyes were from being so upset.

"Hey there, are you sure you want to do this?"

"Do I want to do this, no way, do I think I have to do this, yes sir"

"Remember, you can visit Charlie anytime you want. You know that I love Charlie also and I will keep you updated on his health and anything else that may come up. Don't you worry about him I will give him the best care I know how." He was trying so hard to eliminate my concerns and support what I was trying to achieve.

"I know you will. I just hope he knows how much he has saved my life."

Mr. Cochran looked at me with confusion thinking he must have misunderstood but what he was not aware of was the gift Charlie was giving to me. *By selling him and being as wonderful as he was to me, he gave me the gift of learning how to love and the finances we would need to get away from Pop.*

We walked slowly down the dirt driveway with vines from the overgrown brush grabbing at our legs. When we got back to the barn I led him over to where I had already packed up all of Charlie's tack items including his brushes and food. I reached for the first box of things and handed them to Mr. Cochran.

"Now he loves it when you brush him real good after he has been out in the pasture all afternoon."

"I know," Mr. Cochran said, trying to continue his support.

"His favorite snacks are sugar cubes but remember don't give him too many because that won't be good for him."

"I know," Mr. Cochran said patiently once again.

I lowered my head a bit and said, "I know you know; I just want Charlie to know that I know too."

I paused and then snapped the lead on Charlie's halter and started walking him towards the truck. I could feel his immense power with every step we took as well as his gentle spirit. *This is what I wanted out of life. To have power over my life but be gentle and compassionate. Charlie, an animal, taught humanity where humans did not. This was the final lesson Charlie taught me.*

As we approached the back of the trailer Mr. Cochran gently took the lead out of my hand and led him into the trailer. I walked in beside him again, choking my emotions and told him how very much I loved him and that I would see him very soon. I reached over and grabbed his face, closed my eyes and kissed his velvet nose again. As I inhaled him for the last time I could smell the molasses and grass smell that I loved so much.

I closed the door behind him to make sure that his tail didn't get caught. As I gently touched his tail, I started to remember all of the wonderful things he had brought into my life. I closed my eyes and thought *there is no way you will ever know how much you have changed my life for the better. Thank you for blessing me and please know I love you so much.*

Mr. Cochran placed his hand on my shoulder and with concern said, "Would you like for me to give you a ride home?"

"No sir, but thank you for offering. I think I need some time alone." Feeling like I was going to be ill at any moment, I didn't want to run the risk of getting sick in his truck.

"I want you to know that I get how hard this was for you and I know that Charlie understands it also. You are doing a very brave and mature thing, and I wish you the very best," he said, as he handed me the check.

I appreciated him saying this, but for some reason I felt as if I could just collapse and never wake up.

"Thank you so much," I mumbled, and without looking back I started walking home.

As I turned and walked away, I heard Mr. Cochran's truck start. *Please don't let him drive past me, please go the other way by the school.* When this last thought crossed my mind I could hear his engine roaring beside me as he drove on past. I could smell the exhaust from the truck and once he past my peripheral vision all I could focus on was Charlie's tail waving in the wind as it stuck out of the back of the trailer. Overcome by emotions I fell to one knee and placed both of my hands on the gravel filled ground and sunk my head between my shoulders.

What have I done? Keep your eyes on the ground until they are out of sight.

I was trying to focus on one spot but I could not make out any images through the tears that were clouding my vision.

I no longer heard anything but the sound of the crickets in the pasture beside me and the whisper of the breeze passing by. I wiped my eyes with my dirty hands creating smudges across my face unknowingly. I started down the road back towards our house.

With every step I become more and more angry. The realization was starting to become apparent that the cause for me having to sell Charlie is because of Pop. It made me resent and despise him even more.

If it weren't for him everything would be fine. Mema and Nelly would live with us and I would be able to keep Charlie. I wouldn't have to spend the night with him, scared all of the time that he will sneak in my room at night. I had not only sacrificed pieces of my childhood by hiding from him, but now I had to give up the only thing in my life that I had ever loved.

As soon as I returned home I walked into the house and I could feel the cold air conditioning swallow up my body and I could smell the odor of stale cigarettes. I had worked up a sweat between my anger and the physical excursion on my walk home. I went to find Mom and as usual she was sitting in her chair watching television. I walked over to her and then handed her the check for fifteen hundred dollars.

I looked at her, my eyes and heart filled with determination, and said, "Now, can we please move?"

She looked puzzled and said, "Where did you get this money?"

"I sold Charlie back to Mr. Cochran."

Her face was still, not knowing whether to be thrilled that we had the money or upset because I sold Charlie. Bewildered and concerned she softly looked at me,

"But you loved that horse."

"I still do love that horse, but sometimes when you love something you have to let it go and continue loving it in your heart and appreciate what they brought to your life."

"Mom, I can't live in this town any longer, every day that we are here it feels as if someone is pouring alcohol into an open sore of mine."

With a strong emphasis on my words and without separating my teeth I pleaded, "Is that enough money to get us to Florida?"

"If you're that serious," she said softly. "I guess it will have to be enough. I'll call Uncle Nick and see if he can help."

Thanks to Charlie, my sacrifices, and a lot of begging, we finally moved to Panama City the summer after my ninth-grade year.

CHAPTER 7

HOMELESS TO MODEL

Things were great in Panama City yet the only two things missing were Nelly and Charlie but I knew both of them would be so proud of me. I was at an incredible public school, and I never really noticed a problem with cliques. Mom's job provided enough money to pay the bills, I thought. I didn't understand that moving to Panama City cut off what little financial security she had with Mema and Pop.

I was told that Dad refused to pay child support, and my sister's college tuition cost more than anticipated. Mema and Pop were angry with us for leaving Selma, and they cut off the money they had been giving her too. They were outraged that she had abandoned them.

Aunt Patricia had found a place that was close to school and was in an area of town that wasn't the best but it wasn't horrible either. It was an affordable apartment in a home that is considered a Triplex. I had never heard of this before but it had three apartments in one house. I thought it was the coolest place on earth because it was away from all of the horrible things that happened in Selma. My sister and I had to share a bedroom when she visited us but other than that it was fine. It was about six hundred square feet but was a great place to get started. We lived next door to Lily, Tammy, and Tammy's father.

Lily was sixteen years old and lied about her age so she could work as a cocktail waitress. Her father was dead, and her mother didn't care about her, so she did what she had to do to make it on her own. Tammy and her father lived with Lily to help pay the rent, though they were seldom in the apartment.

Because Evelyn was living with Dad now, Mom seemed to transfer her feelings for Evelyn onto Lily. They became very close and Lily was with us a lot. It was a short, but happy time.

After being dropped off from school one day I walked back to our apartment to find Mom sitting on the stoop crying. She was slouched over just starring at all of our things that were outside of our apartment. As I went running up to her I quickly stopped and looked around in disbelief. I saw our couch, beds, television, kitchen items, bathroom things, clothes, shoes and everything we owned just strode though out the yard. I slowly leaned over and put my hand on Mom's back and whispered.

"Mom, what is wrong, what happened?"

I thought that maybe the house had caught on fire and she single handedly moved all of our things outside so that they wouldn't get ruined. I took a deep breath in through my nose to try and smell smoke and the only detectable scent was pine from the pine tree that all of our things were thrown under. Then Mom finally began to talk.

"The one thing I told you when we moved was that I would not be able to afford living here and because things have been so tough, I have been behind on our rent. When I got home today they changed the locks and all of our things were thrown out here in the yard."

Mom bought a new outfit for work almost every week. Why didn't she have enough money to pay the rent?

It seemed absurd to me, so I began to question her.

"What do you mean changed the locks?" I asked in an authoritative tone and it all started to sink in and I became scared. "Can they do that? This is our house I thought."

"No, it is not our house, it is their house and we pay them to live in it, which is what renting is all about."

Knowing I had to ask the obvious question I came right out with it "does this mean we have to move back to Selma?"

"I don't know what it means."

Not really knowing what to do, I slowly sat down beside her and listened to her weep wondering if all of this was because of me.

I was the one who wanted to move, I was the one who kept on pushing and pushing to get out of Selma. Was all of this because of me?

I sat there quietly afraid to speak.

With a soft sound Mom finally admitted to the issue.

"I am barely making enough to survive and when I had to choose between rent and eating, I chose food because I couldn't bear the thought of us going hungry." Her face was in her hands as she spoke trying not to be seen and only heard.

"Mom, please do not worry because between the two of us we will come up with a solution. We are fighters Mom, and I know we will get through this together." I was trying to think of every encouraging thing I could think of because the thought of moving back to Selma petrified me beyond belief.

She was obviously ashamed of what had happened and didn't want the entire family to know her business.

"Please do not to tell anyone about this, because they will only tell me I was not able to make it"

"Don't worry, I promise I will not say a word," I said, making the motion of zipping my mouth and throwing away the key.

For the first time in our lives, we were truly on our own and as silly as it sounded it felt great. We slowly got up and looked at what we had around us and Mom turned to me, "Well, I guess we need to grab what we can and put it in my car and I will ask Lily if we can keep the rest of our things in her place until we get settled again."

"Sounds good to me."

I started picking up our clothes and shoes and putting them neatly in the trunk. Mom always believed you could be poor as dirt but that was no excuse not to look like a million bucks. There were blades of grass and dirt stuck to them from being trampled on by the people that came to evict us.

Mom went to explain to Lily what had happened and to ask if she could keep our things for a short while. She returned and Lily had agreed to store our things in her house. We spent the next three hours separating necessities that we needed from things we needed to store.

Not having enough money for a hotel room we really had no place to go so we slept in Mom's car for about a week, but beyond that, our lives continued as usual. We would get up every morning and she would drop me off at school on her way to work.

At night, Mom parked in the safest place we knew which was a park that was down the street from where we lived. As we pulled into the park you could see the multiple park benches that were strategically aligned for families to enjoy their time together. It was right on the water and had the most breath taking view at night. We were both exhausted and Mom stopped the car put it in park and looked at me, "well, I guess this is home for now." We were both too tired to care.

"I will take the back seat," and I rolled over into the back seat to start my slumber.

While I was drifting off to sleep I heard the waves slowly glide up onto the shoreline and that sound made me forget about everything concerning.

Every morning when I woke the first thing I would do is inhale as deeply as I could and smell the refreshing morning air. It was better than a cup of coffee. I'd then go to the bathroom in the park to get cleaned up and brush my teeth, and Mom did the same. We made a game of it, pretending we were in another country and had to live this way. I was happier in that car than I ever was living in Selma with that monster.

The car we lived in was a roomy 1978 Chevrolet Impala, and the front and back seats were long enough to hold two people comfortably. We'd lie in the seats, stare at the stars, telling stories and laughing with each other. We were both very happy to be making this new life adjustment. During that first week, we decided that no matter what happened, we would get back on our feet, and we'd never look back.

By the end of the week, Mom had sold a few things and saved some money. We didn't have hardly anything left. Mom did manage to scrape up enough money to move us to a small bungalow in Panama City Beach. I was amazed at how beautiful it was. When we walked through the door it was as if I were entering a mansion for the first time.

"Mom, is this really where we are going to live?" I was stunned at how marvelous this paradise was, new and clean without any roaches or bugs crawling across counters.

"Yes" she said with enthusiasm in her voice. "Do you like it?"

"Like it, I love it!" I exclaimed. I went tearing through the house which didn't take long at all because it was very small. The house was basically one big room that included the kitchen, living room, and eating area, high cathedral ceilings and mauve carpet in all of the rooms except the kitchen and bathrooms. I had my own bedroom and bathroom and so did Mom, we also had a fireplace that was beautiful and the focal point of the entire house! It was built of both wood and stone and was simply stunning.

I went running out of the living room through the sliding glass doors and just stood there looking at the sand in the back yard. Then I noticed a door in the back of the house. I walked down the sidewalk that led to it and exclaimed "Mom, it has a storage room here in the back. We don't really have anything to store but when we do we have a place to put it all!" Then with another breath I turned, *What is that sound?* I stopped my breathing and froze so I could clarify and tune my ears to the sound I thought I was hearing.

Oh my God, is that what I think it is?

I yelled, "Mom, come out here!"

"What is it?"

She took off running thinking something was wrong because she couldn't determine if the sound in my voice was exhilaration or panic. She stuck her head out of the glass doors and stepped down onto to the patio.

"Listen, do you hear that?"

Smiling from ear to ear she could tell by the look on my face that it was something unbelievable.

"Hear what?"

With a laugh in her voice, she closed her eyes and we were utterly quiet.

"I do hear it," she said, and then became infected with my contagious enthusiasm.

"I hear the ocean!" she screamed at the top of her lungs.

She opened her eyes with the same level of excitement as myself and pulled me in for one of the best hugs I have ever had and finally, after all the years of struggle and pain, I felt like we were at home.

A week or so after we moved in, we were so extraordinarily happy. She then told me that she had been speaking with Lily about our things and they were arranging to get them delivered to us.

"Oh really, when do you think we will be getting them?"

I would like to have my bed back because I am so tired of sleeping on the floor.

"We are going to meet in the morning."

We had already been to her place several times to get our bathroom, kitchen, linen items and anything else we could fit into the car. We were sleeping on make shift beds that we built out of the couch cushions. Everything else that was left at Lily's house was too large for the car and would require some type of truck.

Mom continued "Lily has a friend who will let us borrow his truck and even help us move this weekend." Moving on with her sentence she then asked,

"How would you feel if Lily moved in with us?"

Paused and not really looking at me, she seemed to be a bit afraid of my answer. Without even thinking about it I responded, saying, "I think it is a great idea."

Lily and I became very close. My relationship with her was very sibling-like. She made me feel special and let me know that she loved me and cared for me. There were times where we disagreed but were also very protective over one another.

Before the weekend was over Lily, my mother, and I had all of our things finally moved into the house. Lily and I were sharing a bedroom but that was not a problem at all because she usually worked at night and spent the evenings with her boyfriend. We had twin beds and if she were home in the evening we would lie in the room and just talk for hours about life and how our paths had crossed.

When Lily and I were together whatever we did always seemed fun. We used to put on our swimsuits and go to the beach and do what we liked to call "pool hopping." We'd go from hotel to hotel, pretending we were guests to use the pools. We always felt like we were the great deceivers because we got away with it.

I loved living in our beautiful new home with my God-given family. We may not have been related biologically, but we were a well-blended family.

I wanted to let my mother know how appreciative I was for everything we had been through. One day I was awakened by the sound of her banging the pots and pans together as she cooked breakfast. About ten minutes later the smell of pancakes and bacon filled the air which made me smile and jump out of bed.

I couldn't wait to tell Mom how much I loved our life. I went running into the kitchen and threw my arms around her neck while she was cooking the last few pancakes on the stove. "I just want to say that I think it was worth living in the car to be able to live in this incredible home."

As soon as the words crossed my lips I could see Mom's face started to become rigid and appear to look very worried "I am scared, I don't know if we will be able always to afford this place." Her eyes fixed on the stove. I slowly pulled her shoulder to turn her around.

"Don't be so pessimistic; remember we are going to make it through anything." I thought for sure if we could make it through living in a car in the park the rest of life would be just fine. She was working overtime at work and professing to make more money than she had ever made in her life.

"I will do my best to keep all the bills paid but do you think there is any way you could help with my finances?" Surprised by this response I really didn't know how to act. I took a few steps back and started fidgeting with the pancakes that were in the plate on the counter and thought about it for a few minutes.

I have never even had a job and I am only fifteen. I do not even think I am old enough to get one. I was hoping to try out for football like the rest of my friends were doing in the fall. I wanted to go and hang out at the beach and make some new friends over the summer. I didn't know what to do about finances but if this is what I need to do to contribute and help keep this house then that is what I am willing to do.

Picking off a piece of pancake and putting it in my mouth I smiled and said, "Mom, I will do anything I need to do to make sure we stay here."

I was only in the tenth grade, and I wasn't really sure what to do, but I knew I could probably manage a budget.

After looking at Mom's record keeping from her bank account it didn't take long for me to realize that she was not very good at understanding positive and negative amounts. She had more bounced checks and fees for those bounced checks and it was clear that once she started down that negative spiral her spending habits did not change at all. She had been buying clothes, shoes, furniture and things that we just couldn't afford. I was surprised that she could not understand that in order to have certain things that you have to save for them. It seemed that in her mind as long as she had checks to write she had money in the bank.

I did the math over and over again for about a month and then realized that even with Lily paying part of the rent; we needed to supplement our income in some way and fast.

I sat down with them and talked about where we were financially. With an inquisitive look on her face Mom mentioned that she had heard about a modeling agency and thought it would be a good idea for me to go see what I thought about trying to be a model and maybe that would bring in some extra income. I was not old enough to have a "real" job but with parental consent I would be able to make some type of money.

I might be a lot of things but I really don't view myself as being a model but I will give it a shot. Nelly always told me that things are not presented for you to ignore them. They are presented as a gift for you to learn from.

The next day we went to the agency and met a lovely woman named Alicia Pack, who owned the agency. She was tall and stunning and undoubtedly a model herself when she was younger. She walked us into the back of the agency and invited us into her office.

As we sat down she stood up and started to walk around me and looked at me like I was an animal getting ready for auction. She studied me from every angle. I was hoping that I was dressed appropriately and that I was sitting up tall looking like I was supposed to look but this was my first introduction to any type of job and I was more awkward than anything else. I looked at Mom; my eyes betraying my perplexity at what this woman was doing.

She chuckled and softly whispered, "You are doing great."

I didn't want to let Mom down because I knew that she was counting on this to be somewhat lucrative. I continued to sit there stoic as not to have Alicia guess but instead to allow her to study me from every angle.

After about five minutes of silence she finally spoke. "He has a great look," she said to my mother. "I want to take some photos of him to see how he looks in print."

I wonder if she thinks I can't hear. She keeps referring to me in the third person like I am not even in the room.

Mom looked at me, "What do you think?" I was a bit excited about the possibility.

"I am fine with it," I said, not really knowing what I was getting myself into.

Alicia then had a photographer come in and she started giving instructions. He was scruffy with dark patchy facial hair and a baseball hat flipped backwards. He was of a short stature looking a bit disheveled as if he had just rolled out of bed.

Alicia proceeded with her orders "I need some test shots from different angles, face shots and body shots" As quickly as she blurted a command it was as if the guy knew exactly what to do. He asked me to follow him into the next room and without hesitation I jumped up from my chair and started to follow him.

Mom stayed behind to continue her conversation. She stayed posed in the chair with her legs crossed and her arms resting on each side as if she were sitting in a throne. "I will be right here when you get finished so have fun."

As I walked out of her office I looked over my shoulder and smiled at Mom and mouthed the words "this is great!"

The photographer led me into a room that was dimly lit with lamps of different sizes that had oddly shaped lamp shades on top of them. Up against a wall was a huge looking movie screen that he referred to as a back drop. We walked by another photographer that had a smirk on his face. He looked at me like I was a dog being led into a fighting ring.

On our way past him, I overheard the guy make excuses for himself, saying "I am only shooting this guy to pay back a favor I owe to Alicia."

What a jerk to say this right in front of me as if I do not matter.

I was embarrassed and wanted to blend into the wall at that point. Instead, I let myself get angry enough to beat the odds he had started to stack against me.

He asked me to stand in the middle of the lights that surrounded the back drop. I walked out and as soon as I got where he wanted me I heard the words "right there" and about that time a huge flash that startled me.

"Why didn't you give me a warning or something" I asked sternly.

"You should always be ready" as another flash went off.

"Smile, okay now look serious, pull your chin down a little bit, look at the wall, look at the ground and bring your eyes up and try and look at me" That determination was all it took to break the barrier down.

I was very awkward in the beginning but after just about five minutes I began to understand what they were wanting and how I needed to look. The commands continued for what seemed like days. Then out of the blue he exclaimed "Okay, I think we got it. Thank you."

"Sure, you are welcome, thank you," I responded with a bit of a sarcastic tone.

He led me back into Alicia's office where Mom was still sitting.

I entered the door and she turned to me ecstatic "Well, how did it go? What do you think?"

Not really sure how to respond I could only find the words most people my age used and responded with a shrug and a mumbled, "OK". I didn't want her to know that they were making fun of me and that I was totally embarrassed by that guy.

Alicia burst through the door, "He said you were amazing out there and you followed all of his suggestions"

I couldn't believe he would say that. Maybe I judged him too harshly.

"Really, thank you, it was a lot of fun, and he seems really nice," I excitedly blurted back like an immature child.

"What do we do next, Alicia?"

Based on this question, it appeared that Mom and Alicia had discussed some options if things turned out in our favor.

"We will get the film developed and then give you a call. I have a really good feeling about him and I am so glad that you came in today."

We talked on the way home about what I did with the photographer and what she did with Alicia. It seemed that if everything turned out well that I would be under a contract with her and she would help me get jobs. For our financial sake, I was hoping that everything turned out for the best.

I glared out of the window and looked at the vast ocean on our drive home and thought, *I know that Nelly would tell me not to worry because if it is supposed to happen it will and there is nothing I can do to change that by worrying.*

The next evening the phone rang and Mom and I looked at each other with anticipation.

"Do you think it is her?" I was excited if it was and scared at the same time.

"I think the only way we will know is if you pick up the phone," my mother said, smiling both with her voice and with her face.

I was so nervous and so insecure to believe that I could be attractive enough to model.

What if I answer the phone and she tells me I am gross and that for me to think that I should model is a joke? Like Mom said, the only way for me to know is to pick up the phone.

I slowly reached down and quickly picked up the phone, answering it with a breathless, "Hello."

"Hello there, how are you doing? This is Alicia Pack"

She said it as if it were some type of rote greeting.

I tried to think of something interesting, but just blurted, "I'm great, thanks. How did the pictures turn out?"

I couldn't wait any longer.

"Simply amazing," she said without a pause and with the most soothing low tone.

I paused for a quick second and put my hand over the phone, "Mom, she said the pictures were simply amazing."

Alicia could hear the beam in my voice as if I had a great joke to tell and I couldn't get to the punch line.

"Would you mind putting your Mom on the phone?"

"No, not at all; hold on please."

"Mom," I whispered, "she wants to speak with you."

Mom got up and took the phone from me, and all I could hear were a lot of okay's and uh hum's while they talked.

I continuously interrupted her, asking her what Alicia was saying.

"Thank you so much for your call, Alicia, and I am sure he will be thrilled with the news."

She placed the phone into its cradle and screamed, "She said you are incredible!"

We leaped up and started jumping around in a circle as if we were kids playing.

We talked for the next few hours about how Alicia thought I had a great look, and about the opportunities that could be presented to me especially in Japan. I was not sure that I wanted to go to Japan because I had only been in Alabama and Florida. I really didn't want to go to another country by myself.

Alicia told Mom that if I decided to do that I would be able to stay with a host family that was identified by the agency and that I would be safe. I was not convinced. After talking it over we decided it was not only a way to get some extra money, but it would be a good way to help rebuild my damaged self-confidence. I refused to leave the country but I was willing to do catalog work or anything else when the opportunity came up.

We scheduled another photo shoot for the next week and, though I was excited, I had no idea what I was getting into. This photographer was a different guy but he was not as rude as the last one. I felt like I knew more about what they wanted me to do and I got out there in front of the back drop and started going through the poses.

The next week Alicia called once again with good news. "Your pictures were spectacular, and now I think I'd like for you to try some runway modeling."

The only runways I knew of were the ones that planes landed on so I asked for some details, but of course I told her I was interested. She signed me up for a local fashion show to see how I would do. It was a summer runway show being held in the local mall. I didn't care about any of the specifics because I was determined to give it my all.

When I arrived at the mall, Alicia introduced me to another male model named Tony. He seemed like a nice guy and he said something I will never forget: "The way you carry yourself is what sells the clothes. It doesn't matter whether you're wearing clothes from Nordstrom's or K-Mart, people are interested in the clothes because of how they look on you."

He continued to talk to me, but after a while, I was not paying attention to what he was saying because over his shoulder was a room of girls in rollers, men with only boxers on and some woman running around putting clothes together.

This place was the picture of chaos, with people running in different directions and everyone looking like they belonged except me. I was lanky and awkward with bright white hair in the full throws of puberty. I was not ripped and quaffed liked these guys seemed to be.

It was incredibly exciting to see all the activity in the room as people scurried around with clothes, putting on makeup, fixing hair, and hearing the occasional zipping sound of duct tape ripping off of the roll. Suddenly a man walked through and yelled, "Twenty minutes, people!"

I looked at Tony to see what to do, and he said the show started in 20 minutes. I began to panic, my thoughts were numerous and scattered. Part of me wanted to flee and the other part of me wanted to see what the experience would actually be like.

What am I doing? Have I lost my mind? Why would I think I would be capable of doing something like this? What would Alicia say if I told her I wanted to back out? I have to get over this! Just suck it up and do what needs to be done!

I asked him about what to wear, and he said look for clothes with your name on the tag, which would also have the information about what change the outfit was.

I had no idea what he was talking about; I looked around, found my name. It was attached to a pair of plaid shorts and a purple tank top.

I hate tank tops and the color purple even more.

Behind my name was the number one, so I assumed I needed to wear it only once. I went behind a curtain where there were several other guys changing clothes and as I opened the curtain a pungent odor that smelled like a homeless person that had not bathed in months hit me in my face.

Oh, gross, I thought. I took a deep breath and held it, trying not to inhale too often because of the horrible odor. I timidly undressed and held the clothes that were tagged with my name close to my body. As I scanned the room looking up hoping not to be noticed by anyone I realized the extent of my insecurities. My body didn't look anything like these guys, in my opinion.

They all looked as if they had never eaten an ounce of fat and that they lived in a gym. Most of them were in their twenties and I was certain I was one of the youngest there. Once I had the tagged clothes on I quickly ran out from behind the curtain and then took a deep breath.

With my hands on my knees a heavy-set women came up to me and said, "Honey, you're up next," as she pulled the tag off of my shirt.

I said okay and took a step up. As I glanced over my left shoulder, all I could see were people everywhere, and I felt a moment of panic, *I can't do this* I thought. Then I heard Alicia announce "Our next model is wearing . . ." and I never heard anything else she said but I did see her lips moving. I was panic stricken.

At first I didn't move, and then I saw Alicia smiling at me. She covered the microphone with one hand and mouthed the words "come on" and motioned for me to walk on stage. With a cheery tone I heard, "Show them what you have on."

That subtle reminder was all I needed. I knew I could do anything I set my mind to. I put my other foot on stage and held my head high and literally felt my knees begin to tremble.

You can do this just keep on walking and try not to look at anyone. Remember one foot in front of the other, one foot in front of the other.

I continued to chant as I made my way down the runway. Once down there I turned a few times, and by the time I made it back to the middle of the runway, people were yelling and screaming with delight.

For a minute, I thought someone well known must have come on stage, and everybody was excited about that. When I turned to walk back, however, I realized I was the only person out there.

Could that have been for me? I thought in disbelief.

I made it to the steps of the runway and looked over my shoulder to see Alicia wink her approval at me. I stepped carefully down the step backstage and followed the path designated for us. The same little heavy-set lady met me and ordered me to get dressed for my next change. I asked her what she meant.

"Honey," she said dryly. "You've got to do that three more times."

My eyes must have looked like saucers because she smiled and said, "Don't worry. You did a great job. Didn't you hear them cheering for you?"

"That was all for me?"

I couldn't believe all that applause and cheering had been for me. All I had done was walk down the runway displaying the clothes I was wearing. She looked at me funny and said, "Who did you think it was for?"

I finished the show and was simply amazed at how incredible I felt once everything was finished. I enjoyed what I had done and knew it was the kind of work I could really get into. I did a few more shows that summer and the more I did, the more it was evident that the first experience was only scratching the surface of this business. Most people I worked with were either self-absorbed or horribly insecure. They were using their looks as a vehicle to maneuver their way through life. The reality was, there were always people more beautiful, exotic or with a fresher new look. It was a constant cage of insecurity. So many of them were damaged because they sought acceptance based on their looks not who they were as people. I knew I was damaged but I was not sure if I had begun to fall into the same trap.

About two weeks before the start of my eleventh grade school year, I received a call from Erik, one of the guys I modeled with that summer. He was an older model, and he told me he had a good friend named Terri who was looking for someone that could work a few hours during the evenings. He said he'd immediately thought of me for the position because I was so personable and easy to talk with.

I asked him what type of modeling it would be and he said it wouldn't be modeling. I would be a retail person who helped people pick out clothes and ring them up at a register. I was supposed to let Terri know if I was interested. By the time the phone hit the cradle, I was dialing her number. She asked me a few questions, and then asked if I was sixteen years old.

After a quick pause, I assured her I was, even though my birthday wasn't for three weeks. I was hoping the job wouldn't start before my birthday.

Before we hung up, we agreed to meet so I could tell her more about my experience. Since I had none, I decided it would be a brief conversation.

I went running to Mom's room to share my good news. I was going to have my first job, and I'd be able to help with the bills until we could get some money in the bank. She was thrilled and for the first time felt that we truly could conquer anything. I explained all of the details of my call and she listened intently and agreed that she would be more than happy to drive me to meet with them.

I arrived for my interview and followed the instructions Terri had provided to me over the phone. I walked up to the front counter and asked if I could see the store manager and about that time she came walking around the corner. She was a strong looking lady, classy and smart which is exactly what I had pictured her as. My first thought was that she reminded me of Stockard Channing, who was one of my favorite actresses.

She came up introduced herself and immediately started the conversation. "You look great, Erik has told me so much about you I feel like I should just go ahead and offer you the job. Let's step out into the office in the back and see if you have any questions. I explained most of it to you over the phone," she continued as we walked towards the back of the store and through a door that led down three stairs into a store room.

"I really don't have any questions for you I am just so happy that you called me and I appreciate you considering me for the job." I was afraid I was starting to sound rehearsed with my speech. I had been practicing what I would say the entire drive up to the mall with Mom.

"Great, I do have one more person I would like for you to meet if you have the time." I was not prepared for this. I had only rehearsed what I would say to her not to someone else. I didn't want to blow this opportunity for me or Mom.

"Sure, I would love to meet them." I lied but I didn't want to tell her no. She excused herself and walked up the three stairs and through the door back onto the sales floor. She returned about two minutes later with a lady she referred to as the assistant manager. "This is Cathy, and she helps me manage the store on my off days." Cathy seemed harmless enough so I stuck out my hand to shake hers "delighted to meet you."

The next words out of her mouth surprised me. She looked at Terri and resentfully blurted "Are you going to hire another air-head model type to work here?"

It was as if I didn't even exist to Cathy when she said that. I was angry that she would judge me and not try to give me an opportunity based on my looks.

Terri encouraged her to talk to me because she believed I would be a big help. "Weren't you referred by Erik?" I thought that she already knew the answer to this but to clarify things I still responded

"Yes he did," I said half smiling but yet still incredibly nervous. She followed that with "Why do you want to work for her?"

Why do you have to be so rude I thought before answering?

"Because my mom and I need the extra money, and I need to learn a lot about fashion and style this summer."

Intrigued by my answers she went on to ask, "Where is your dad?"

"He lives in Mobile somewhere but I am not sure where." Trying still to be respectful, I felt like she was crossing a line.

She ended the interview and walked back to Terri and said, "Okay this time, but let me pick next time."

When Terri came back she told me to bring my social security card and drivers license with me on Monday when I started. "So I got the job?"

"Yes, if you want it."

"Oh my gosh, of course I do. Thank you so very much."

I was so excited I didn't even find out how much my pay was. I just ran out to the car to tell Mom the great news. She was so excited for me and started asking a million questions. "How much money will you make per hour?"

"Um, I forgot to ask," I said laughing.

"When do you start did she say?"

"Yes, I start on Monday and they will train me on everything".

"Mom, I don't know if I can handle the cash register though."

"Don't worry. She said they would train you, right?"

I thought for a second, "Yes she did."

"Well, then there is nothing to worry about."

I arrived Monday with my learner's permit and my social security card. I was very nervous because I knew I'd have to tell the truth about my age. When I told her, she just winked at me and said no problem because she was going to let Cathy pick the next new hire.

"I'll use your permit number until you get your license, but let's keep it quiet. Is that a deal?"

"Oh, yeah, it is definitely a deal."

The job worked well for me, and I was delighted to see the cash registered supplied the change amount so I didn't have to figure it myself. I still practiced transactions in my head, but it was nice to have an accurate back up. I was sixteen and making minimum wage, but it was still enough to help with the household budget.

CHAPTER 8

Ending The Cycle

It was July fourth and we were in Gulf Shores to celebrate. The local beaches had fireworks and every year we would watch the beautiful explosions that lighted the sky. I still recall the scent of salt and sulfur in the air mixed with the tranquility of hearing the waves lap against the shore. It was intoxicating listening to of the crowd's reaction with every colorful aerial display.

At fifteen, I had very little interaction with Mema and Pop, except during holidays. This particular trip I was feeling a bit different. I was older and had developed a stronger sense of independence and confidence thanks to living in Panama City. I knew that there was nothing that Pop could do to me even though we were staying with them, as we always had. Mom was excited to see Mema and I was hoping to see my cousins and stay as far away from Pop as possible.

It was around nine in the morning the day after we had arrived when I heard voices coming from the other room. The conversation was not loud enough to hear the words that were being exchanged but it was loud enough to know it was Mom and Mema. I lay there staring up at the ceiling hearing the beautiful sounds of the morning. The birds were singing outside the windows and I could see the light from the morning sun dancing all over the room.

I slowly sat up on the side of the bed, looked out the window and saw that it was another clear and sunny day that was perfect for hanging out at the beach. I took in a deep breath and relished in the realization that there is nothing purer than the smell of the ocean air first thing in the morning.

I pushed up onto the mattress to lift myself to the tan tile floor. The tiles were old and had never been replaced since the house was purchased twenty fives years ago. Some of them were chipped and cracked at the corners. They were tan asbestos tiles and back then no one knew they were dangerous. When my bare feet touched the floor I could feel the cold shoot up through my legs cooling me off. I had started to sweat from all of the sun that was beaming into the room.

I went to the den to join the conversation that I couldn't quite make out. I saw Mom and Mema weren't there, but then knew they must have been in the kitchen. As I walked through the den still in my bare feet I passed Mema and Pop's door and I was thrilled to see he was still sleeping. It was rare for him to still be asleep because he was usually the first person out of bed in the morning.

I passed through the door in the kitchen and saw them sitting at the kitchen table drinking coffee. They were up and dressed for the day. The smell of coffee in the morning is one of the best smells to wake to. The day was starting out simply perfect.

"Good morning," I said as I walked to the sink to get a drink of water. They briefly paused in their conversation "Good morning," and went right back to the story. I sat down and joined them for a moment trying not to interrupt. They were planning the menu for the day. Everything seemed to always revolve around food. They would spend hours and hours trying to plan a meal for lunch, spend a few more hours cooking the meal and then get the dishes cleaned up in time to start dinner. The food was always great but it would get really boring after a while to spend so many hours talking and hardly anytime enjoying the beach and festivities that were going on for the holiday.

Uninterested in getting involved in their planning, I leaned over to Mom and whispered "I am going to get into the shower," and walked back to the bedroom. I hated having to shower here because I couldn't lock the doors. They were folded like an accordion when you opened them and were not designed for security.

Once the door would hit the frame you could hear the magnets click against the metal frame and the sound let you know that the door was closed. I knew that Pop was still asleep and with Mom and Mema in the kitchen it seemed like the perfect time to go ahead and get my shower in for the day.

I turned on the shower and undressed. It usually took a few minutes for the water to get warm, so I folded my clothes and placed them on the edge of the sink while I waited. The walls in the shower did not meet the ceiling so anyone could stand on a chair and watch you take a shower. In fact, one of our favorite games as children was to pour a pitcher of ice water on top of whoever was in there and then laugh and take off running and hope they couldn't figure out it was you.

The typical response we got was, "Just wait till you take a shower."

I could see the steam start to fill the room so I pulled back the shower curtain to expose the very basic shower. It had a cement floor with a drain in the middle, a pipe that ran up the cinder block wall and then split into two pipes. The pipe on the left had a blue shower knob for cold water and the one of the right had a red shower knob for hot. They looked like they were off of a garden spout from outside, circular with spokes in the middle. Both of them had broken so they were difficult to turn. The shower head was rusted and sprayed water all over the shower instead of in a controlled stream.

I placed one foot inside of the shower and then the rest of my body followed. I slid the curtain closed and then soaked my body with water. It felt great rushing all over me and it was the best way to wake up. I was about halfway through my shower when my mom yelled, "Mema and I are going for a walk to the boat landing if you want to join us when you get out."

I was startled out of my relaxing moment. With her yelling like this it meant that Pop was awake. I didn't want to be in the shower with just him and me there alone. Trying not to panic I said, "I'm almost done if you two don't mind waiting."

"No, if you're almost done then you can most likely catch up to us. We'll see you when you get there."

Please don't leave; give me a minute.

I started rushing as fast as I could. I had not yet washed my hair and I had soap all over my face. I knew I had less than five minutes to rinse, dry off, get dressed, and get out of the door to get out of harm's way.

I heard the door shut behind Mom and Mema, so I began to rush. My heart dropped into my stomach, and I became almost paralyzed as I heard the bedroom door slide open. I yelled, "Mom?"

I didn't get a response so I thought my mind was playing tricks on me. I tried to calm down. I began to imagine where they were on their walk and what the best route was for me to catch up with them as I hurriedly turned off the water. I opened the shower curtain and the clothes I had placed on the edge of the sink weren't there. Maybe I'd left them on the washing machine just outside the bathroom door. I was trying to remain calm and give myself the benefit of the doubt.

I looked to the wall where I had placed my towel on the towel rack and it was there so I pulled it off and dried myself as quickly as I could.

If I can just hurry up and get out of here I know he will not do anything because he just woke up.

As I put my hand on the door handle, I heard the sound of a belt buckle rattle. I could feel the blood race out of my face and my finger tips started to get numb. This sound was chillingly familiar. I knew exactly who it was and what it meant. I just had to decide what to do. I was sick and tired of his crap, and I wasn't going to tolerate him raping me again.

I opened the door and there stood that nasty old man, very naked, stroking himself. *You sick bastard, I wish you the best of luck this time trying to violate me.*

I almost felt as if I was hoping he would try something. I was furious until I remembered I was also naked. I needed my clothes and I looked to the right on top of the washing machine but they weren't there. *Where in the hell were my clothes?*

I looked over his shoulder at the dresser and still didn't see them.

He leered at me and said, "I sure have missed you."

Not even acknowledging what was said, I stoically looked at him with hatred in my eyes. My voice much lower than before and gritting my teeth I asked him

"Where are my clothes?"

He didn't even pretend to hear my request

"I was thinking we could play around like old times," he said.

"I don't think so. Mom is waiting on me."

I noticed he had his left hand behind his back and that he was holding something in it but I couldn't make it out.

"Once again, I am asking you where my clothes are."

He moved his left hand slowly out from behind his back showing me my clothes. He then threw them across the room and the only way for me to get to them was to pass beside him.

"They won't be back for at least an hour." His voice was not making me scared, it was making me angry.

I felt my panic rising a bit as I realized he was right. The walk to the landing took about twenty minutes, so it would be at least a forty-minute walk and they usually sat on the dock for at least a half of an hour listening to the birds and watching nature waking first thing in the morning.

This time was different. I had been away from him long enough to know that what he was trying to do is wrong. I was frightened but not because of him, instead because I was willing to fight. If it meant I would die trying to protect myself, then I was willing to accept that consequence.

He reached out and grabbed my arm. He was extremely tall and weighed about two hundred and twenty pounds, which was mostly muscle. This man could lift an engine out of a car by himself. I was all of one hundred and thirty pounds.

One minute I was scared and the next minute I wanted him to attempt something. I was determined that he would not violate me again.

Before I had a chance to plan an escape, he threw me on the bed. I hit the bed and bounced onto the tile floor. Startled for a brief moment, I couldn't decide what to do. The only option I saw was to hide. I began crawling on my hands and knees to get under the bed. Feeling again like an animal being hunted, I moved as quickly as I could. That's when the fun began for him. He always seemed to love the challenge of the chase.

"You know you can't get away from me, right? I have you all to myself for the next hour."

I swear there was glee in his voice.

I thought, *you may have me here for the next hour, but it's not going to be quite as pleasurable as you think.*

The worst thing that could happen was he'd beat the shit out of me and have to explain it to my mother. This time I was going to hunt him and try and watch him try and get out of it.

I crawled under the bed and was almost to the other side before he grabbed my leg and dragged me across the tile floor until he could see my face. I had lost my towel when I fell onto the floor from the bed. I was now naked and felt the grit on the tile floor scraping my stomach and chest and the jagged edges of the broken tiles ripping my skin as he pulled me. I grabbed the bed frame, trying to keep myself under the bed, but he was just too strong.

My legs were kicking as if I were trying to come to the surface to get air. I kicked him in his ribs and again in his shoulder. I was kicking anything I could come in contact with fighting harder than I had ever fought before. He eventually got me out from under the bed and pushed me on my stomach.

He had his hand in the middle of my back pressing all of his body weight against me. Between the hard surface of the floor and the pressure of his hand and weight I was struggling to breath.

He leaned over and folded his arm and placed his elbow across my shoulder blades and looked down towards my butt and tried to put his penis inside me. I raised my head up and hit him as hard as I could in the face with the back of my head. I could feel the bridge of his nose crack as my head smashed into him.

"You little bastard," he started screaming.

Stunned, he slowly reached his hands up to his nose. As he pulled them away he saw the blood. The power of my blow made me a little dizzy. I couldn't get my balance but at that point I knew it was life or death. I had never fought him like this before. I started thrashing all over the floor trying to get out from underneath him. I could feel the corners of the tiles from the floor cut into my skin and the sand start to scrape sores on my hips.

He grabbed me again and pulled me from the floor, pinned me to the bed, and whispered into my ear, "This is exactly what I like, wrestling you to get what I want."

This time I was not going to tolerate it. This time I was either going to die trying or I was going to kill him. I had the control regardless if he knew it or not.

Well, buckle up, asshole, and get ready for the wrestling match of a lifetime.

I could feel him getting more aroused the more I struggled with him lying on top of me so I became subdued, moving less and acting submissive.

"Now you know what is best for you," he said.

"Yes, okay. What do you want me to do?" I asked quietly knowing he would eventually start letting his guard down.

He got to his knees and began crawling up toward my face with his penis coming toward me. "Now, suck my dick."

I slid down to his groin as if I was going to do what he asked. I sheepishly looked up at him and I opened my mouth and without a second thought, I bit down as hard as I could, bringing my teeth together viciously holding on like a pit bull. I had bit down so hard I could start to taste his blood in my mouth.

He doubled over and screamed, "You fucker!"

I was pinned between his legs so he could not reach any part of me but the top of my head. I then reached up beside my ear, through his legs, released my bite and pulled on his penis like I was the anchor in a tug of war match. With the loudest scream I have ever heard from a man he rolled off just enough for me to get away.

I loosened my grip with both my hands and my mouth. He was flailing around trying everything he could to get me off of him. As soon as I released my grasps I immediately fell back towards the door. I could have easily went running out of the room but not this time.

Leave, just leave, he is not worth it. I tried telling myself.

I was stunned! I was actually standing up for myself against him and had control. For the first time in my life he was in a place where he should be scared of me. I was going to inflict on him what he had inflicted on me my entire life. I looked around me for something to hit him with, but the only thing I could find was an antique chair that went to a dressing table. I hated to harm the beautiful chair on something that was such a piece of garbage as he is, but it was the only thing I could get that would be effective.

I picked the chair up and hit him with all my strength across the back. The chair back separated from the seat upon impact, and he fell face down on the bed, moaning.

"I want you to know I hate you for everything you have ever done to me. You are cruel and disgusting and not worth my time. I hope you rot in hell." I quickly grabbed my clothes. I looked back to see if he was getting up.

My eyes met his, and I swear I was looking at the devil. He was up on his knees facing the door with blood saturating his lips and teeth from where I had hit him in the nose.

"Boy, I swear I will kill you." I knew he meant what he said.

He began to move slowly, and I started to feel terror again. I knew I had to get out of there. I pulled on my shorts and headed for the open door, hopping the whole way, struggling to put on my shorts.

As I hopped past the television, I noticed my car keys lying on top. We'd driven my early sixteenth birthday present Dad had given to me. It was a candy apple red MG convertible.

I quickly grabbed the keys and threw my shirt over my shoulder. I looked back and Pop was hurrying toward the door.

Oh my God, if he gets to me I know I am dead.

I ran as fast as I could to my car and jumped inside. I knew I was breaking the law because I only had a learners permit. However, under the circumstances, I praying a cop would show up.

Sitting now behind the wheel, I stuffed the keys into the ignition. I looked up and he had startled me. He was at the driver's door, banging on the window. Then the naked old fool ran around the front of the tiny car and I knew he was going to try and open the passenger door. I reached over and rapidly locked it to prevent him from gaining access.

He came back around to my side, trying to punch a hole in the convertible's top to get to me. I turned the ignition, pushed in the clutch, and accidentally put the car in first gear. When the car moved forward, I realized my mistake.

He jumped on the hood of the car and yelled at me, "Remember what I said I would do to you if you ever told anybody about this!" He banged on the hood of the car. "I will *kill* your mother if you drive away."

I paused, but only for a second, put the car in reverse, and punched the gas. As I reached the next house, I saw Mom and Mema on their way back to the cabin.

Mom stood in front of my car, and I stopped and rolled down the window. She looked at me and said, "What do you think you are doing?"

Terrified he was still trying to get to me I looked in the rear view mirror. I saw the old man walking back inside. I knew it was now or never.

"Mom," I said softly. "I can't explain, but I am so sorry."

Not letting that go for an excuse she started to yell "Sorry, what are you sorry for? What did you do, what happened? Tell me something! Don't you drive away from me young man, do you hear me?"

I rolled up the window and she continued to yell at me, "Wait, you are not a licensed driver. You get back here, right now . . ." I heard her words and saw her mouth moving but nothing was registering.

I didn't really know what to do, so I just kept driving to the end of the street.

Should I turn around and go back? What if Mom is really mad at me when I see her again? What if he tries to kill her? I can't stop now, I have to do something about him. He is crazy and if he does try and kill Mom, I need to let people know.

I got to the end of the street and the only direction to turn to get you out of the neighborhood is left. If you were to turn right it would take you down to the boat landing where they were earlier.

I was not sure where I was going but I knew I could not undo what had just happened. The adrenaline that was pumping through my veins was starting to subside. My body was beginning an assessment of the damage that was inflicted. I felt the sting of the abrasions that were left on my stomach and chest. The blood from the cuts on my hips where he had dragged me across the jagged tiles was starting to coagulate and stick to my shorts.

I reached up to the rear view mirror and pulled it towards me. My lip had been busted when he grabbed me by my head and shoved my face to the floor. I re-adjusted the mirror and slowly placed my hand on top of my head. I could feel the heat radiating off of the huge lump that was left from head butting him in the nose. As much as the lump hurt, it felt good to know that this time, I reclaimed some more independence and stood up for myself.

The road had nothing on it but a few houses. It was long and winding and if I stayed on it long enough it would lead me to the highway to take me out of town. I didn't know how to get back to Panama City from there and I didn't want to try. I started to recall what had just taken place.

If I were Mom what would I do right now? I would go inside and ask Pop what just happened. I am sure he would be able to explain away the bloody nose to then make up a lie about my behavior. He would try to be a hero, plus show them how great he thought he was, hunt me down and bring me back home.

That thought quickly started to echo in my mind.

What if he did try and find me, there would be nothing keeping him from killing me, making it look like an accident. He could drown me; drive my car into the water with no one knowing the difference. I have placed myself in the worst possible position to truly let him kill me and get away with it. I have seen how calm and collected he can be on the outside, while on the inside he is a raging lunatic.

What have I done! I should have stayed and made him explain to Mom what he tried to do to me. If I had done that he could have killed both of us. No, I did the right thing I just need to stay hidden from him until I can figure out what to do.

Trying to decide what my next steps were, I remembered Dad was on vacation in a town about forty five minutes away.

I know he wouldn't find me if I were with Dad. Mom wouldn't allow that and I couldn't imagine her even calling him asking if I were okay. Should I go? More importantly, would I be caught?

Finally, I decided I didn't have any other choice. I couldn't go back to the cabin.

Immediately on my left was the Corner Store. This little store had been there for years, and the owners knew my whole family. They knew all of the divorces, affairs, and trouble my sister had always gotten into.

I pulled into the parking lot made of oyster shells. I could hear them clank against the undercarriage of the car as I rolled to a stop. I thought it would be best to park for enough away from the store, so my car couldn't be seen if they drove by.

I jumped out of the car, looked down the street to see if anyone had followed me. There was complete silence in the air. Not only did I not see any cars, I couldn't hear any movement. I could feel that things had changed at that moment.

I slipped back to the front porch of the store and as I was walking to the door, I realized the only way to keep him from doing this to me and others was to tell. I had to tell someone.

I walked by the ice machine that was directly beside the front door. I saw a pay phone, *who can I call just in case he finds me and tries to kill me? I want someone to know what just happened and what has been happening my entire life.*

I picked up the receiver, knowing I'd call the only person I knew who would believe me. She wasn't in my family, but she knew me better than anyone. She would know I was telling the truth, and she knew everyone else well enough too.

I went to dial the number; I felt in my pockets and realized I didn't have a penny on me much less enough money to make a long-distance phone call. Then I remembered about collect calling. Evelyn had started doing this when she called Mom and she explained what I needed to do. I picked up the phone and pressed zero.

The operator came on the phone and said "May I help you?" I was shocked that she picked up the phone so quickly.

"Yes, I'd like to make a collect call," I said hesitantly.

"What number would you like to call?" Her voice was cold and distant, but I was elated because it really worked!

I gave her the number, and realized the time and feared Lily would likely still be asleep.

"Hold please while I ask if they accept the charges."

Not sure what that meant I patiently waited and started to pray, *Lord please let her answer the phone, please let this call wake her up if she is sleeping.*

Before I could go any farther into my prayer the operator interrupted. "I will connect you now."

I was thrilled!

With a sleepy tone Lily said, "Hello Grant, what's going on?"

As soon as I heard her voice, I breathed a sigh of relief.

"Lily, I need your help, and I don't know what to do. Please call Dad and tell him to come and get me," I said.

"What's going on, Grant?" she asked, her voice laced with concerned.

"Pop tried to hurt me again," I knew that I had to get her attention so that she would call Dad. I couldn't find the words to tell her he had been sexually violating me for as long as I could remember. I could only tell her that he has been hurting me since I was a child.

I continued to glance down the street to see if anyone was coming from the cabin. I crouched down between the door to the store and the corner of the ice machine.

"Lily, did you hear me?" She was there but I could tell she wanted to ask a million questions but respected me enough to know I was scared.

"Grant, I will do anything for you," Lily said. "What number should I call?" I didn't have a number for him. I didn't know where to find the number but I knew that Lily could find out.

"I don't know. He is on vacation in Destin," I said, my voice edged with desperation.

"Where in Destin?" she asked.

I told her he was in a condominium called San Destin and asked her to tell him to pick me up at the Corner Store in Golf Shores. "He knows exactly where it is. Please tell him to hurry because if Pop finds me, I'm really afraid he will kill me."

"Why don't you just call the police?" I could hear the fear in her voice.

"Because, I just need to get away from here as quickly as possible and I don't really know what to do but I know I will be safe with Dad and Samantha.

"Okay, sit tight and call back in about ten minutes so I can try and find them." I had given her such brief information but I knew that if anyone could find him she could. I could see the clock on the wall in the corner store and I paced from the front door to the edge of the street for what seemed like hours waiting to call her back.

I couldn't wait any longer. I looked up at the clock and it had been exactly ten minutes. I went back through the same steps as I had before and called her collect. To my surprise it worked exactly the same way the second time as well.

"Lily, did you get in touch with him? I know I didn't give you very much information but I am just so scared." Not trying to alarm her but wanting her to know how serious I was about getting in touch with Dad.

"I did, and I spoke with him. He asked me a million questions and I just repeated myself letting him know I didn't have any details and he would have to ask you. I told him you were at the Corner Store in Gulf shores and he wanted me to tell you he was on his way."

I couldn't believe it. I finally felt like I was not going to die. I knew everything that had happened to me would be coming to an end.

I fell back against the wooden exterior of the store and slid slowly down the wall. I felt relief as she continued talking to me, helping me calm down.

I had to interrupt her "Lily, I have to go inside the store now because if he drives by and sees me sitting outside then I am afraid of what he might do."

I didn't want her to think I was not appreciative for what she had just done but I needed to stay in survival mode.

"I will give you all of the details later but I am sorry I have to go. Thank you for calling Dad and I want you to know, I love you."

"I love you too and we can talk later. Call me and let me know when you get to a place that you feel safe."

"I will."

I hung up the phone and made one last glance down the road. I saw a car in the distance this time but it didn't look familiar.

I ran inside and the clerk behind the counter greeted me like they always did. "Good morning, how's life treating you today?"

I froze looking at them emotionless. I didn't say a word so it was obvious they could see by the blood coming through my shirt and the bruises on my face that something had happened that answered their question.

With panic in my voice I asked, "Do you have a place I could sit while I wait on Dad to pick me up."

He knew who Dad was because of the nasty divorce he and Mom had. It was her goal to make sure everyone knew how horrible he was and how much of a victim she had become.

I knew he didn't know how to answer me and without taking their eyes from my now stained shirt he said, "Sure that isn't a problem."

"Do you mind putting me in a place where no customers can see me? I want to be able to look out onto the store though, so can you think of a place where I can see others and they can't see me?"

I didn't want to go back into their office because if Pop came in trying to convince them it was okay for him to take me, I didn't want to be trapped. I begged that they put me somewhere so I could see who was coming and going. I didn't want to be caught off guard in case Pop did walk in, I could run and escape.

He led me back to the butcher area, behind the display cabinets. "If you crouch down here beside the sink and the wall, you can see people before they see you."

He said this as if it were a common place where he hung out while business was slow.

"Thank you so much! Please, if anyone comes in here looking for me, don't tell them where I am. The only person I want to know is Dad." I begged.

"No problem but do you need me to call a doctor or something?"

He was looking at me as if I were about to fall apart. Knowing I probably needed the medical attention, I didn't want to run the risk of being in the hospital emergency room and having the doctors tell Mom to come and pick me up.

"Please don't. Dad will know what to do and I just need to have him pick me up."

I squatted down in the corner where he suggested and he was right, I could see the door and almost every area of the store. I saw him walk over and tell someone else I was there and as he talked I could see her look at me with a furrowed brow.

She stood up on the tips of her toes to get a better look and nodded to the guy and walked away. He came back about ten minutes later and checked on me and offered to get me something to drink but I just wanted to disappear.

I pulled my knees into my chest and never took my eyes off of the door. I could smell the odor of raw meat all around me but I was having a hard time distinguishing if it were coming from me or the butcher cases.

As I sat there and considered all of my escape options just in case Pop did come into the store I could feel myself starting to doze off. The rush of adrenaline was truly subsiding and I was beginning to feel safe. I cautiously sat down on the floor with my back against the wall and my feet out in front of me so I could stay awake.

About an hour later, with my drowsy eyes still permanently fixed on the door I saw Dad arrived. He came into the store and I could see the concern in his face. I couldn't believe that he had actually come to help me. I was so relieved to see him. I could feel my body start to shake with anticipation knowing that this would be over soon. I saw him walk up to the front clerk and ask for me. When I saw him point to my hiding space, I jumped up, ran to meet him, and gave him the biggest hug I had ever given anyone and thought it was finally going to be alright.

Dad peeled me off and looked confused, "What in the world happened to you and what is going on."

His voice was authoritative but concerned at the same time. I couldn't tell if he were upset with me or angry out of fear.

"Dad, please let's get in the car and I will tell you everything I promise."

He put his arm over my shoulder and we walked out to the car. As we passed by the clerk that had kept me safe I paused for a moment.

I stuck out my hand to shake his, he slowly reached toward mine and said, "Take care of yourself and if you ever need to come here again you certainly can." I was certain he was just being kind.

We walked outside, I saw my stepmother, Samantha, waiting in the car, and she gently waved to me.

I don't know why, but at that point I began to sob uncontrollably. I guess it was a release because I was getting away from Pop and I had been so frightened. Dad said he would drive my car and Samantha could drive his. I didn't care who drove what, I just wanted to get away from Gulf Shores.

Dad and I got into my car and pulled out onto the road, and he asked me again what was going on. Cautiously I questioned, "Dad, I need for you to be open-minded when I tell you this and I don't want you to get mad at me. Do you promise?" Looking at me very puzzled, he glanced my way still trying to keep his eyes on the road. I could tell he wanted to know what I needed to tell him but was scared to hear what it must be. His eyes were darting from the road then back to me and with uncertainty in his tone he finally responded after what seemed like hours, "I promise." That was the confirmation I needed to tell him everything but I was scared to tell him the truth. *What if Pop were right and all of the things he told me about how people would react to me telling the truth was accurate. What if he does hate me for this and think I am a sick pervert? What will I do if he pulls over and drops me on the side of the road or worse if he takes me back to the cabin?*

I had to trust that he would hold true to his promise. I couldn't hold it in any longer, "Dad, Pop has been sexually molesting and physically abusing me as far back as I can remember. Today he tried it again, and I was able to get away." His eyes stopped darting back and forth only focusing on the road in front of him. His body language was very awkward and I could tell he would have preferred to be anywhere in the world right now instead of sitting beside me. *Is he going to say something? Oh, my God, Pop was right; he isn't even looking at me anymore.* Afraid to say anything else I just sat there and mimicked his behavior. Eyes focused on the road but on the inside feeling like I was the most horrible person in the world for burdening Dad with this type of news.

Finally the silence was broken. He broke his gaze to look me right in the eyes and say, "Why did you lead him on?"

Oh my God, I thought, *Dad does think I'm a freak. He thinks that all of this is my fault, that I initiated this.*

Turning his head back to the road he only said one other sentence for the rest of the trip that I will never forget "I don't think I am ready for Samantha to know all of this yet so let's just keep it quiet for now," Seething with disappointment I just stared at him. I know he could feel my glare penetrating the side of his head. With my mouth ajar I couldn't help but rant in my head. *He is ashamed of me and I didn't do anything. How could I have led him on when I was only three years old? I don't even know how to lead someone on and why, of all people, would I want to lead on Pop?* Knowing it was useless to continue the conversation any further I stopped glaring and turned to look out the passenger door window. *So what if Samantha knows? Does it make me a bad person or does Dad thinks it makes him look bad that I am not perfect? Does he think that now that he has this new life that I am just a burden? I think Samantha would be supportive for what I did back there instead of blaming me for what happened. How could he have possibly just said what he did to me? There is no way that I asked for this! I thought he would wrap his arms around me and protect me from any further abuse but instead he is keeping me at a distance. I really thought he would keep me safe but I think instead he hates me for telling him. What did I do to cause this and why is this happening to me? Most other people's parents would do anything in the world to keep their children safe but my parents are far too worried about themselves to care for their kids. What am I supposed to do if Samantha asks me what happened? Is he expecting me to lie? I can't lie to her because she will know and then I will lose her trust.* I continued beating myself up verbally for the rest of the trip and not another word was uttered between us.

When we got back to their condominium we pulled through the gates and parked right in front of the unit they had rented. I did not pay attention to the surroundings because I was too busy starring at the ground wishing I could just disappear. Dad turned the car off and as I reached for the door handle I looked out the window at Samantha parking beside us. As she reached down to turn off her ignition she looked right in my eyes. Her look was nothing but sincere and deep concern for the reason I had called them. *What am I going to do if she asked me what happened?* I paused to let her out of her car first and after she shut her door I opened mine. She waited for me to get out of the car and I walked in front of her and started walking up towards Dad who had already made it to the front of my car. As I expected the first words out of her mouth hit me like a brick wall, "Please tell me what was going on." I immediately looked up at Dad as if to say, you handle this because I will only tell her the truth. Without even giving me the opportunity to say anything Dad reached out and gently grabbed my arm and looked over his shoulder to Samantha and said, "It was no big deal. He just overreacted. Let's go watch tennis."

She knew me better than Dad did and refused to let it drop but didn't want to pry because she was uncertain of the conversation we had on the way. Her tone was insinuating she wanted to help and responded "Chuck, are you sure? He looks a little bit pale. How did he get so bloody?" She wanted to get Dad alone so she could continue with her questioning and proposed that I get cleaned up, "Grant, why don't you go upstairs and take a shower and a nap while we finish watching tennis? You look exhausted."

"I'm not really tired," I mumbled and then it hit me. *I left all of my clothes!* Knowing I could fit into Dad's clothes even though they would be a bit big, I was frightened to ask. I was afraid that he would not want the germs of someone that was as disgusting as me, to get on his clothes. I guess my blank look was all Samatha needed to understand what I was concerned about, "Chuck, go pull out some of the clothes you brought so he can have something to wear when he gets out of the shower." Dad looked at her as if to say, I can't believe you just asked me that and stomped off reluctant to honor her request.

"I am so sorry I don't have any clothes with me. When I went running out I didn't think to grab any extra." I wanted to tell her everything so badly.

"Would you like something to eat or a snack?" She was trying so hard to console me without asking questions.

"If it's not a problem, I'm starving," I said, not knowing if the hunger pangs in my stomach were from anxiety or lack of food. She turned opened the refrigerator and pulled out some fruit, cheese and grabbed some crackers, "Here you go, this should hold you over until dinner. We are planning on having your favorite, fried shrimp." I was so hungry that everything sounded good but there is nothing in this world better than Samantha's fried shrimp. Wide eyed, I said, "What time is dinner then!" I was starting to feel relaxed and normal again. She was making small talk while I ate the snacks she had prepared and did everything she knew to do to make me comfortable.

Dad came back, handed me some clothes and off I went to the shower. I had a full stomach; I was feeling safe and wanted to do all that I could to go un-noticed. After the shower, I curled up on their bed and feel asleep for about an hour. I awoke to the sounds of an announcer chattering about the commercial break. I was hoping the previous part of my day was just a nightmare. I looked down at my bare chest and saw the scrapes and cuts and my head was still pounding. I knew it was real. I slowly got up, put on the shirt Dad had loaned me and walked out into the den area where they were rooting for their favorite tennis play Boris Becker, the seventeen year old from Germany.

For the rest of the afternoon, I gazed at the TV, pretending to watch tennis because I wanted to belong somewhere and feel normal and loved. I knew I didn't belong with my mom, but I didn't believe I belonged with Dad either.

On my drive back to Panama City after being with Dad, I dreaded what I had to do next. *I know she is going to want answers on why I left Gulf Shores so abruptly. I am going to have to explain why I drove away and why I didn't call her to tell her where I was or what I was doing. I have to tell her what horrible things he did to me.*

I am petrified about doing this. All my life that old man had threatened to kill her if I told anyone what he did to me. I know it is time to call his bluff. I have to tell somebody all of the details because I want this bastard put behind bars for the rest of his life.

The entire forty five minute drive from Destin I couldn't focus on anything but what I was going to say to Mom once I saw her. I turned the corner and saw our little house and I immediately got butterflies in my stomach. I knew she was there because as I pulled into the driveway I could see the light on in the kitchen. *I have no idea how she got back but I am sure she is pissed at me for leaving her stranded which is not going to help.*

I got out of my car, took a deep breath, and headed for the front door. I tried to imagine what my mother would do once I was done telling her all of the specifics. I tried not to have any expectations because I didn't want to be disappointed and I didn't want to get too excited about the possibility of never having to see him again. *What if she called to tell him what I had done? What if she didn't believe me? This was her father, and I am not sure if her loyalty will be for him or me, her son.*

I opened the door and didn't see her at first. When you walked into our beautiful small house, it was an open, airy room that included the kitchen, dining room, and living room. The only doors in the house were to the two bedrooms and bathrooms.

As, I approached the kitchen counter, she opened her bedroom door and said, "Well, it's nice of you to show up." I could tell by her sarcasm she was already upset with me.

The look on my face must have been convincing. Of course, it was helped by the bruises all over my face and body.

Her tone changed immediately and she asked, "What's wrong?" It was time for me to tell the truth. I had convinced myself that no matter what happened I had to tell her everything.

Lily came walking around the corner and startled me. I did not expect her to be there. "Hey there, welcome home," she said as she came walking up to me, kissing me on my cheek. Just her being there made everything so much easier. I knew she would support me and help me tell Mom what I needed to tell her. After she kissed me she gently touched the bruises on my face and sighed and softly whispered, "Come on now, we need to tell Mom what happened."

"Thank you so much, I am glad to be back, it was an interesting weekend and you're right." I didn't want to chicken out so I knew that as interested as she was in knowing what was going on, I had to get the first sentence out and the rest would come easily.

"Mom, I need to talk to you about something," I said softly. "It has to do with Pop." Looking at Lily as the words came out of my mouth, she nodded and smiled with approval as if to say perfect job.

"Okay, with frustration in her voice, what is it?" she asked. I knew that regardless of how she took it I had to do this for me. I couldn't hold back I had come too far and I knew Lily was there to help me through it.

"I don't want to make you mad, but I need you to believe me and trust what I'm telling you is the truth." If I could get her to trust me then we could work through the rest.

"I promise I will," she said. "Please tell me what's going on." She was oscillating between being sincerely concerned and overtly frustrated.

I pulled the bar stool out from under the counter and sat down. She walked to the end of the counter, fumbling in her purse. Lily leaned in beside me and put her hand on my back to let me know she was there.

"Mom, your father tried to rape me in Gulf Shores." My voice betrayed my edginess.

She pulled out at cigarette from her eel skin case I bought her for Mothers Day, slowly put it in her mouth, pulled out her lighter and lit it, pulling in a huge inhale of smoke. As she exhaled, she gave me a strange look and said, "I can't believe he did this to you too." I sat up for a moment paused wondering if what I just heard her say was accurate. I looked at Lily and she had the same mystified look.

I jerked toward her. "Too? What do you mean too? Are you telling me you knew he had done this before? Why would you put me in a situation with an abuser?" The room started spinning and I was feeling nauseous from the smell of her cigarette smoke. I couldn't believe that all of these years of torment and fear were something she could have known about. It was impossible to believe that she knew what he was capable of.

"Well, he did it to me too," she said blandly.

"So the fact that he did it to me will be overshadowed by knowing he did it to you first?" I asked with astonishment. "You knew he would do this all along?" I was mixed with emotions not knowing if I should punch her or just walk out.

"No," she said. "I didn't think he'd do it you. I thought he only did it with little girls, not boys." She thought it wouldn't happen to me but it was both Evelyn and I that would stay there alone. I know for a fact that she was alone with him on several occasions. If she thought he only did this to girls, how is that an excuse?

I couldn't hold back anymore I asked, "Do you think he did it to Evelyn?"

"I'm not sure," she said slowly as she inhaled another lung full of toxic smoke. .

"You might want to ask her," I said sarcastically

She just looked at me and finally said, "What do you want to do about it?" I couldn't tell if she really cared but I saw anger in her face that I had never seen before. Through the plume of smoke that surrounded her face, I could tell she was not upset with me but she was angry with Pop. I was going to push forward and tell her everything I wanted and everything that I needed from her.

"I have two things I'd like do," I said purposefully. "One, I want to live with Dad and get therapy. Two, I want to turn Pop into the police so he can burn in jail." I waited cautiously for her response to both of my demands ready to debate. That was it; I had laid it all on the line.

She took another drag from her cigarette and said, "I will do whatever you would like. I just don't know why you would want to go and live with your Dad. If you want Pop to be arrested then I will see what I need to do to have that happen but if you go and live with your father I can't stay in this house. His child support is the only reason why we can afford it." I expected her to find some level to guilt me on but since I was the one that understood the expenses I was surprised that she would say something like that. She might need to make some budgetary adjustments to accommodate for me leaving, but she wouldn't have to lose this house that meant so much to us.

I wanted her to understand so I accepted her concerns and said "Mom, I know you don't want me to go and live with Dad. I really haven't ever had a true male role model in my life other than Pop which can't be healthy. I don't know if living with Dad will change anything for me but it is something I feel strongly about." She put out her cigarette, and put her hand on her hip, "If you feel that strongly about it maybe there is something I can work out with your Dad." I was so surprised! She was actually willing to let me go and live with him without too much of a fight. I looked up at Lily a bit confused. I didn't know if this meant I needed to go and pack my things or if I needed to wait and let her talk to Dad. I was scared to be excited and also scared because it was such a huge change. Dad and I didn't have the best relationship and we had not lived in the same house in years.

"Mom, thank you for understanding but what if I get there and I hate it, would you let me come back?" I sounded as if I couldn't commit but she was so incredible.

"Son, if you want to come back of course you can, if you want to stay I will get use to it. Now, let's not dwell on that. I need to make some calls so we can get all of this moving." I jumped up from the counter and ran around the bar. I waded through the smoke cloud that was surrounding her and hugged her whispering, "I am so sorry, I didn't mean to cause problems." I could hear her start to cry, "It wasn't you that caused these problems it was him for doing what he did, I am sorry you have gone through so much." She pulled me away from her and asked, "Do you mind if I call Uncle Nick so he can help me with some things?" I thought that she would want to let him know so he could talk to me or they could work together to confront Pop. "No, ma'am not at all if you need me to talk to him I will."

"I think you have had to say enough tonight." She left and walked into her bedroom to take the next steps to help support me.

CHAPTER 9

OPRAH WINFREY SAVED MY LIFE

Uncle Nick, mom's oldest brother, was a Methodist minister. She trusted him completely because he was one of her strongest Christian connections. She confided in him about the abuse I had gone through and shared with him the stipulations I had made about moving in with Dad, therapy, and prosecuting Pop.

Uncle Nick gave her the name of a friend who was a therapist working with several congregations as a counselor for children. He assured us that Doctor Henderson would be a great fit for me. She called the Doctors office the next day. Unfortunately, his office was in Pensacola which meant it was an hour and a half trip one way from our house to his office but she was not concerned if it was the right thing for me.

I believed she really wanted to get me some help and in doing so it helped ease her guilt. Of course her ulterior motive was that she didn't want me to move in with Dad because she would lose my child support.

We made the long drive to Pensacola to meet the man Uncle Nick thought so highly of that could help me. We pulled into the parking lot and I leaned forward and looked out of the front windshield. The building looked like it was built in the seventies. It was a five story building made of tan concrete. The windows were tinted so dark it was impossible to see inside. Overall it seemed like a nice enough place. We got out of the car and walked up to the building marquee to see what floor Dr. Henderson was on.

Mom turned to me and said "Well, he is on the third floor. Are you okay to go in and talk with him?" It seemed as if she was not comfortable with me telling him so much about my past. She was visibly more nervous than I was but I didn't recognize why. Knowing what I knew about her abuse from Pop, I was starting to realize I was opening a vault in her mind that had been closed for years. Anxious to get the help, I looked Mom in the eyes and enthusiastically said, "Yes, let's go, I can't wait to meet him and understand more about me. I am a little bit scared though, I hope he doesn't think I am crazy." Mom laughed at my comment, "Honey, there is no promise about that, after all, you are a part of this twisted family." Laughing nervously together we walked up to the dark tinted door and went inside.

The smell of disinfectant wisped around the heavy, solid dark brown door as we opened it to reveal the waiting room on the other side. It was small with dark carpeting and dim lighting. Chairs lined up against the wall facing a receptionist that was hidden behind a frosted glass sliding window. There were two other people sitting in the room. I began to feel panic, *what if they know I have been sexually abused? I wonder if they were sexually abused or if they are crazy? Were they waiting on someone that was back there or are they here to see the same guy?* We signed in and walked over to the farthest corner of the waiting room beside the very dark tinted windows. I sat and waited as patiently as I could and neither of us said a word to one another. I was so nervous by the time my name was called that it startled me. I stared at the lady standing in the doorway with the clipboard in her hand. *What will everyone think if I get up? Will they think I am crazy or that I have issues? Will they find anything out about me from the Doctor or will they talk about me behind my back when I am out of their sight?* I slowly got up from my chair and walked shamefully toward her with my head down wishing I was invisible.

She led me down a short hallway to the first door on the right. It was heavy and dark wood and maintained the same continuity as the décor in the waiting room. She knocked and I could hear a muffled sounding "Come in." She opened the door and part of me wanted to run the other way. The other part was so very thankful to have this therapist help me understand why all of this had been happening to me for so long. His office had the same sterile smell as the waiting room. Once I walked into his office and saw him, I began to feel a bit more relaxed. Across from the door was an entire wall of nothing but windows that looked out onto a street. There was a sofa to the left, and along the back wall were his desk and two chairs in front of it and a bookcase behind them.

I didn't know what to expect from a therapist. When he looked up, I was surprised to see how young he was. As I approached the desk, I couldn't decide if I was nervous or excited to tell someone all the horrible things that had happened to me. I was secretly hoping I would have a kind of world-altering revelation and forget all the pain and the embarrassment I had suffered.

I got closer and he stood up and stuck his hand across the desk. I cautiously raised my hand up to shake his. "Nice to meet you young man," he said in a quiet and calming voice.

"Nice to meet you too," I said cautiously.

"Why don't you tell me why you're here and how you think I can help you?" He pointed to the chair that was in front of his desk showing me where I should sit.

At first I didn't want to say a word so I just sat there. Afraid he would judge me or that he would tell me it was my entire fault. *Regardless of the outcome, he is here to listen.* I repeated in my mind over and over. *I need to do this for myself and find out what this therapy stuff is all about. What would Nelly say? She would tell me that the reason why God put me here in front of this man was to tell him everything I could about Pop and what he had done to me. She would then ask me "What's the worst thing that could happen?"*

That was all I needed. For the next hour, I talked non-stop, telling him everything I could remember and how upset I was about all the things that had happened to me. He was feverishly taking notes as I talked. I went into detail about the physical, mental and sexual abuse. We then talked about sexual abuse in general, my feelings about the mistreatment I had been through, and what I needed to do to understand the impact it could have on me. As he continued through statistics of abuse victims that became drug addicts, underachievers, hospitalized in institutions and repeat sexual offenders. I realized that this guy had no idea who I was or what I was about.

Feeling like I was just placed into a category of victim instead of being heard as a person I became disinterested in what he had to say. *He is stereotyping me instead of listening to me. He is telling me what I am going to be like instead of getting to know me to help me understand myself.* No longer interested in his elaborate summation, I looked at him with a piercing glare and directly asked "What does this have to do with me?"

Obviously shocked by my directness stopping mid sentence and with a long pause he commented, "I thought you wanted to know about abuse."

"I do but not as it relates to the rest of the world statistically, I want to know what I need to do to heal the pain!" I said sternly as I moved to the edge of my chair.

He looked at his clock, "That will be a great place to start next week. This first meeting is to really lay the foundation of what we need to cover and get an understanding of the outline for therapy." He said this as if to be relieved that an hour of time had passed because my straightforward manner seemed to startle him and make him uncomfortable.

He stood up and walked across the hall to the receptionist and asked that she get my mother in to speak with her. As he came back in his office, he asked that I go back out into the waiting room because he needed to speak with Mom. I got up and walked out the door and passed her in the hallway. She asked "So how do you feel?" I could tell by her voice that she was deeply hoping this was the last time we would ever need to be there and that this would only take one visit. "Fine I guess." I didn't really know how to respond without going into great detail. "Great, I will see you in a few minutes," and she disappeared into his office. She came out about ten minutes later with tears in her eyes. Afraid he had told her I was a psychopath or a lost cause I grabbed her by her shoulder and leaned to look into her eyes, "Mom what's wrong, what did he say to you?" She just said, "I am so sorry," looked down at the ground with her eyes unable to make contact with me and walked to the car.

As we drove home it was dark outside. She had her window cracked, eyes on the road smoking a cigarette blowing the smoke out of the car through the crack as she exhaled. We said very little and I kept wondering if I was in trouble now that the secret was out.

I stayed quiet, but inside, I was freaking out. *If there is something that is going to happen to me I think I have a right to know it. Did he say I provoked this? Did I somehow cause all of this to happen to me and if I did what do I need to do to stop it? Does she hate me for telling him everything? Am I a bad person for wanting to get some help dealing with this? What if my friends find out, what will I say to them? Do I have to tell my teachers?* I continued questioning myself the entire ride.

Once we got home, I asked one question, "Can I go back next week?"
She said, "Without a doubt."

Because Mom couldn't leave work early my appointment was his last one of the day. I couldn't wait to talk to him again, and, fortunately, there was no one waiting when we arrived, not even the receptionist. He opened the door and walked out with his other client and said their goodbyes. He looked over at me, "Are you ready?"

Unlike the last time I was there, I jumped up and said, "I'll see you in about an hour," to Mom and practically ran across the waiting room. The week had been nice because I was finally telling someone the deep dark secret of my life. I was realizing that it was not something I had done to myself. Pop was the one that was sick not me. I finally was feeling good about myself.

The doctor looked at her and said, "If you want to get some dinner, feel free. You don't have to wait here." He gave her some ideas of places that were close by.

Mom smiled and said, "Thanks, I might just do that." I knew she was probably starving because she had not had time to eat dinner before leaving Panama City.

He held the door for me and I went straight to the chair I'd sat in last week. I was ready to have a conversation that was about me this time and not about statistics. He sat behind his desk and asked how things had been going.

"It's been great. Thanks for asking," I said hurriedly. I was ready to get to business and talk more about what I needed to do to get over what had happened.

I heard the lobby door close and assumed Mom was going to grab a bite.

He stood up and said, "Why don't we go sit on the couch so we can both be comfortable?" I had already started in my conversation so I thought nothing of it. I stood up and didn't miss a word as I walked over to the couch. Rambling on about how I was afraid of what Mom must have been thinking when we left there the last time.

He turned off his lamp and turned on one beside the couch. Oddly, the lamp beside the couch was very dim, but I didn't question it. When I sat down, he sat right beside me with his writing pad in his lap.

Stopping my chatter I was not sure why he sat so close to me on such a huge couch. I moved away from him a little, feeling somewhat uncomfortable. I also noticed his left arm was above me on the couch, but I thought I was just being paranoid. He was a professional and Mom trusted him to be there alone with me and he was a Christian, according to Uncle Nick.

Finally, he said, "Now, where did we stop last week?"

"I don't remember, but can I talk about my plan?" I was anxious to tell someone about getting Pop arrested and wanted to tell someone to make sure that I did it correctly.

"Of course," he said sympathetically.

As soon as he said that, his left arm dropped to my shoulders. I couldn't tell if he had placed it there to make me feel more comfortable with him or if he placed it there unknowingly. I froze, feeling my panic rise but said nothing.

"You know, I've been thinking about you since last week," he said, letting his hand slide from my shoulder to my chest. Not sure what he meant by that I tried to ignore the suspicious feelings he was evoking within me. I continued, "I have been thinking a lot about my talk with you too." I was trying to keep the focus on the reason why I was there but I couldn't help but sense that he was trying to get intimate with me. I couldn't decide if he was testing me, if he was trying to see how I would react or if this was a new way to teach me how to know when things get inappropriate.

In my mind I began to realize he was doing this because he could. I thought , *you sick pig. You're hiding behind your profession just so you can manipulate little boys.*

My mind went back to all the abuse I'd suffered from my family, and my uncle recommended this man. *Did Uncle Nick know he would do this to me? Why would he put me in a position to get abused by someone? This is so sick, and I am stuck because we both know Mom just left to get some dinner. Will I go to jail if I try and get away? Will he try and get me committed telling everyone I need hospitalization as he explained last week?*

"Can I make a suggestion?" he asked softly, unbuttoning the top button on my shirt. His breath smelled like the peppermint he just popped in his mouth before sitting down beside me.

I was frozen, looking directly in front of me, feeling trapped and afraid. My arms felt like they were being held down by anvils as he used his body weight to rub up against me to lower himself to one knee on the floor. I couldn't believe this was happening again.

"How about you write your grandfather a letter about how you feel."

I saw his lips moving, but didn't hear anything he said. I felt him undo the last button and then my shirt was completely open and he was going for my shorts. He first undid his belt buckle and unzipped his pants exposing his penis. I tilted my head back on the couch feeling such hurt and anger. *God, what are you doing to me? Why is all of this happening? Last week I had told this man about all my weaknesses, and now his hand is on my stomach while he is getting sexually aroused.*

I finally snapped out of it and grabbed his hand. I put my face in his and said, "You are a sick pervert, and I can't believe you're doing this."

He said, "Isn't this what you like?"

Appalled, I jumped off the couched and started buttoning my shirt back up. He went to reach towards me but he was struggling to pull up his pants that had fallen around his ankles while he was getting up. I pushed him back and ran for the door.

"Where are you going?" he yelled. "Your mother left. Didn't you hear the door close?" *He had planned this all along*, I thought to myself.

As I opened the door, I glanced up and saw someone on the other side. It was Mom. She said, "Is everything all right?" with a mystified tone.

"I think it's time to go," while I finished buttoning my shirt. She didn't question me and grabbed her purse and threw it over her shoulder. I went over to the elevator and pressed the button to go down. "What happened in there?" I was afraid she might have been a part of everything Uncle Nick had planned so I was scared to tell her. I looked at her as the elevator dinged and responded, "Nothing out of the ordinary," and I walked in and pressed the "L" button to take us to the lobby.

We headed for the car. As we shut the doors, Mom again said, "What happened?"

I said the first thing that popped into my head, "I think I need a female therapist." Afraid to press any more she turned the car key and started the car and we went back home.

After visiting several therapists, I realized the common theme was making sure I didn't have suicidal tendencies. Every new therapist always asked me if I'd ever felt suicidal, and I always said no. What I wanted to say was, "Why in the hell would I want to kill myself because of what that bastard did to me? I wouldn't give him the satisfaction of dying because I always thought he was trying to kill me."

As a teenager, one of the therapists I had interviewed recommended group therapy with people who had also experienced sexual abuse as an alternative to one on one therapy. I wasn't sure she understood the magnitude of my abuse, but I didn't feel I should close the door on an option. Like Nelly always told me, "Doors are open for a reason, it is up to you to walk through it or not." I wanted to walk through every therapeutic door that opened because I hated feeling like a person unworthy of emotional love, only capable of being screwed and tossed aside.

I signed up for her group therapy session hoping it would be what I needed. The experience was one of the worst I've been through. After we introduced ourselves, the first woman who spoke talked about her fear of being on a crowded highway. She discussed at length the stress it gave her and how proud she was that she had driven to therapy by herself. We all listened with fake intensity. I asked her how far away she lived, thinking she must have come a long way, but she said I live about five miles away.

I immediately thought *what a mess!* She is scared to drive a car five miles, and I'm supposed to share my sexual abuse story with her?

The next person said she was there with her husband, who wasn't in the room, and as I glanced around, I realized I was the only male who would be talking.

The married woman continued, telling us how she and her husband had sexual issues because she had been abused by her father. She said her husband thought she was just somewhat shy and afraid to get naked, which made their sex life impossible.

I really didn't want to hear anymore about their sex life, and, frankly, I thought discussing it with the group was inappropriate. More people introduced themselves and discussed what I considered insignificant phobias such as a fear of veterinarians, husbands, ropes, and talking. The more people talked the more out of place I felt and the more closed off I became.

When the therapist asked me to speak, I just looked at her, wondering if she was totally crazy for telling me I should be there. I told her I didn't feel comfortable talking about it and she passed to the next person. All I wanted to do was get out of there as quickly as possible but I didn't want to draw attention to myself so I was going to wait for the right minute to excuse myself to go to the bathroom but not come back.

She divided us into pairs and said we should talk with each other in what I considered a situation that was way too intimate. This was the perfect opportunity. While we were all being paired up, I raised my hand told her I needed to run to the restroom real quick. Horrified at what I was being asked to do I walked into the bathroom, splashed water on my face, waited for about ten minutes and ran out to my car.

The one thing I learned from group therapy was it wasn't the place for me. I never felt comfortable in a group situation confessing to total strangers that I didn't know or trust. Later she called me asking what had happened and I just reiterated that I didn't feel comfortable telling complete strangers about my life.

This experience caused me to restrict my feelings and keep them internalized. I believed I was the only person who had been sexually abused in the manner I was. Therapists kept telling me I was a victim, and I kept saying nothing was my fault. I refused to feel guilty because Pop was an abusive monster.

I decided it was time take a break from therapy and even looked into what suicide involved. Because I was feeling like no one would be able to help me and I would never amount to anything based on all of the statistics everyone had told me regarding victims of abuse.

Being a planner, I felt I had to look into all aspects of suicide in order to do it correctly. In studying carbon monoxide poisoning, I found you need to sit in a car in a closed garage. Since we didn't have a garage, I couldn't even consider that option. Next, I thought I might use a gun, but feared I'd miss and then have to explain to everyone and end up in another endless cycle of therapy.

I contemplated a drug overdose, but I had no narcotic prescriptions and didn't want to break the law by buying illegal drugs. The only other method I knew about was slitting my wrists, and I wasn't sure I could stand the pain of that.

I guess I must be really gullible because I saw a report on the news of a man who died from dehydration in Florida and decided that might be a good way to kill myself. I'd simply quit taking in liquids. Living in Panama City, I had no trouble getting to a hot beach, where I could sit and let my body dehydrate. I don't think I truly understood the concept of dehydration.

Looking back, this seems like a hilarious episode in my life when in reality it was a desperate attempt to rid myself of the grief from my sexual abuse. I also felt I should at least try since my therapists had all felt it was important.

After my time in the sweltering heat and sun on the beach, I returned to the house. I was starving and desperately thirsty. I decided to fix a lunch with no liquids and turned on the television for company. When I heard the announcer say Oprah Winfrey was coming on, I went in to watch. Mrs. Rouse, my English teacher, had told me about Oprah. I felt very close to Mrs. Rouse, who was also African-American.

Mrs. Rouse was a single mother and a wonderful teacher. She provided an excellent role model for all of us, and I admired her very much. Her daughter received a scholarship to Harvard University, which I thought was incredible. Knowing what Mrs. Rouse had said about Oprah, I decided it might be beneficial for me to watch her show.

I knew Oprah was an African-American pioneer in the broadcasting industry. She had taken her talk show into syndication and was a huge success. Her business empire was growing, and she had basically set her course herself.

I have always felt a real connection with African-American females, probably because of my relationship with Nelly. I think it was especially true at this time in my life. They made me feel safe and being with these women was comforting for me. I felt that sense of safety as I went in to watch Oprah's show.

I was waiting for her to introduce her guests and see what unusual phobia she would discuss today. When the show came on, I saw a beautiful African-American woman sitting in a chair quietly announcing to the world that she was a victim of sexual abuse. I couldn't believe what I was hearing. How was it possible that Oprah had been sexually abused?

As she continued the story of the abuse that was inflicted on her by her uncle, I suddenly realized sexual abuse is not something that can be lumped together as single cause for therapy. Each case is individual; each person suffers something different.

I gave up my poor attempt at suicide and grabbed the gallon of water out of the refrigerator and listened with rapt attention to the rest of Oprah's show. As she talked about her life, I began to relate to the story and slowly understood more about myself than I ever had. The more I listened, the more I wanted to hear. I wanted to learn about more people who had suffered abuse, but had come out of it as whole persons and were living happy, successful lives.

I headed out to the library and started my research. I went directly to the card catalog and looked up sexual abuse. I found a lot of books about criminals and the rapes they had committed, child abuse, the abusers' past and the dysfunction abuse caused, but I could not find out anything on sexually abused people that were successful or functional.

I stuck to it and eventually found presidents that were cross dressers and had sexual identity issues, sexually transmitted disease and all about homosexuality but nothing on successful survivors of sexual abuse.

Then understanding dawned. Once again, Oprah was a pioneer. She was the first person I'd ever heard discuss sexual abuse publicly and say you could move beyond it. From that day forward, I began searching for myself in the midst of everything that happened in my life.

CHAPTER 10

TAKING NOTES AND CLEANING HOUSE

Samantha came into our lives when I was thirteen; Dad started coming around more. I thought it was because he was missing me and wanted us to have a stronger relationship. I realized pretty quickly that he had a dilemma. He had fallen in love with someone and wanted to take their relationship it to the next level, but felt guilty about me and my sister.

She and Dad met while working together after my parents divorced. They married about a year into their relationship. She was very impressive to me however; my impression was tainted because Mom had always said she was a slut and a bitch. When I met her, that wasn't what I encountered at all. Samantha was tall with beautiful green eyes and brown hair.

Dad told us about Samantha, and I realized he wanted Evelyn and me to approve of him being with her. Ultimately, it was my mom who disapproved. When Evelyn and I returned from a visit with Dad, she told Mom he had a new girlfriend, my mother was furious. She called Samantha a whore and a bitch and said she couldn't believe Dad would date someone who had sexually transmitted diseases.

I wondered how Mom knew these terrible things about someone she had never met. I also wondered why she was getting so upset and angry.

I was in bed later, just falling asleep when my mother came into my room. She gently rubbed my forehead and hair and asked me what I thought about Dad's new girlfriend. I told Mom I thought Samantha was nice. Then mom asked if I thought Samantha was prettier than she was, and I took the safest choice. I said, "No, of course not."

The next morning, Mom spread the news to the rest of the family, and with every phone call, Samantha became uglier and more of a whore and more contagious. I even began to believe what my mother was saying because she was so convincing. Mom had mastered the art of manipulation and took pride in turning everybody against a person.

Dad picked me up one day and took me to lunch alone, and I thought it was odd that he'd drive more than two hours just to have lunch with me. When I asked about it, he told me he needed my opinion about something. He took the opportunity I'd presented and pulled over to talk to me.

"What would you think about me getting married?" he asked quietly.

"I think it would be a great idea. Nobody should have to live alone," I said. "If you find someone you care about, I think it would be important to get married."

"You're very wise for somebody so young," Dad said.

I shrugged and said it just made sense to me.

He asked me not to tell Mom because he wanted to do that. Based on her reaction to the news of him getting a girlfriend, I was certainly not going to tell her this news.. When he told Mom, she was angry and began raving about what a whore Samantha was and how other people had told Mom that Samantha was sleeping with everybody in Mobile. I was shocked to hear that because I didn't think Mom had any friends in Mobile.

Despite Mom's protests, Dad and Samantha got married on September 4, 1982, which was my birthday. It was a simple wedding at the home of Samantha's mother, with just Evelyn and me as witnesses.

I spent the entire day confused about what I should be feeling. I didn't know if I should be happy for Samantha and Dad or upset for my mother because Dad had married a horrible person. I'd never felt anything like this before. I stood on the steps beside my father with a big smile on my face because he was so happy and tears in my eyes because this truly meant the end of my family.

When we returned home, Mom had very little to say to us. She didn't ask about the wedding, and she treated us like we were traitors because we'd gone to it. I was left wondering what I should do and whose side I should take when the truth was, I didn't want to take anybody's side.

Mom continued telling us horrible stories about our new stepmother, and, as time passed, I began to believe them because Dad seemed to pull himself further and further away from Evelyn and me. It occurred to me that Dad had put his life with us behind him and started over. He never expressed any interested in what was going on in my life, and we eventually stopped talking to him. We'd hear from him on holidays and occasional spontaneous visit throughout the year.

Originally, I was excited about Dad's anniversary being on my birthday, but as I grew older, I realized Dad chose the date to replace the celebration of my birth with the celebration of his new life.

When we visited Dad and Samantha, it was incredibly uncomfortable. Dad overcompensated by buying us a lot of things and trying to keep us busy. I knew he was trying to balance his new life with his old but it was not working out so great for he and I.

I decided to embrace Samantha instead of taking my mom's tainted view of her. I think she is one of the most incredible people in my life still today. She has been a sounding board, a friend, a parent and always a huge supporter of me.

One day while visiting, she came in and said, "In an effort to better understand what you've been through, I have poured through literature and read every book available to me. Based on everything I have learned, you should be dead."

I was stunned, wondering what she meant.

"Between the divorce, your sister, the abuse and your life, you are the perfect storm," she said bluntly.

I was laughing until I noticed she had tears in her eyes.

"How did you do it?" she asked quietly.

I didn't have an answer for her then, but if I were asked that question today, I'd have to say things changed for me when Samantha came into my life. She helped me put into practical use all the things Nelly had taught me.

She was loving and accepting and didn't act one way at home and another way in public. I had grown up thinking the most important part of a person was good looks and a good public persona. Getting to know Samantha and her family taught me what a healthy relationship was and how you should relate to people in an honest manner.

I adored Samantha's father, Rodney. I kept my distance from him in the beginning because I was afraid of most men around Pops age or had a grandfather type role, but he eventually became a good friend. He was funny, caring, opinionated and, most importantly, respectful. This was something new for me. He cared about what I had to say on a subject and gave me solid advice with no underlying schemes for personal gain.

Rodney's relationship with Samantha's mother, Victoria, was very loving and nurturing, and it was the first time I'd ever seen parents who put their kids first in their lives. They gave me a great example of what it was like to live in a healthy, loving family and, for the first time, I began to have hope for my future.

They lived in a wonderful house that looked like it should be featured in *Homes and Gardens* magazine. Sitting on top of a hill, it was a lovely corner lot with a beautifully manicured lawn. In back there was a brick fence that matched the brick on the house.

There was a pool inside the fence with a slide and a diving board. When I was there, I felt like a happy kid and wondered if this is what other kids feel like. It was like an amazing oasis.

Victoria's green thumb was really evident as you walked from the back porch to the pool. The wonderful scent of the flowers surrounded you, and you couldn't help but enjoy the designs she mapped out with the incredible colors.

When I walked across the patio through the fragrant pathway, I always looked back to the glass doors to see what was happening. I probably did this out of habit. With my family, it was done to place myself strategically out of the path of danger. But with Samantha's family, every time I looked through the doors, all I saw was a group of people who loved one another. You could actually feel it just being around them. It was the first time in my life that I fully understood what that meant.

Stepping across the threshold into the den gave me a sense of serenity, and the wonderful aromas inside would make my mouth water. Victoria was always in the kitchen cooking some type of seafood meal for the afternoon. Gumbo and fried shrimp were my favorite, and she always seemed to have one or the other of these dishes when I was there.

The best place to sit was on a barstool at the kitchen counter. That way I could enjoy seeing everyone gathered around, talking and laughing about old times, friends, and family. I felt like a spectator looking at a live taping of the perfect family.

The things they talked about were completely new to me. They were not gossiping or seeking to hurt people by discussing their problems behind their backs. These conversations were about sharing pride in accomplishments, no matter how insignificant they were. The greatest part was that their pride was genuine and heartfelt. Samantha's sister was in law school, and they talked about how smart she was and how amazed they were with her intelligence. She would humbly oppose their amazing support and kind words.

I greatly wanted to be a part of this family, and thanks to Dad I was. I felt like I'd had a start on a brand new life. I secretly wanted to call Victoria my grandmother and Samantha's sister my aunt, but I couldn't. Even though I was an outsider, I felt accepted and valued as part of the family.

I was terrified they might learn the disgusting things that had been part of my childhood and would hate me. My biggest fear was they would tell me never to come to their home again. As a result, I was careful about everything I said to them, thinking about every word that came out of my mouth.

I was falling in love with this family, and I wanted to be protected by them. I realized that it was the kind of relationships and dynamics I wanted to have when I grew up and established my own home. It wasn't perfect, but it was a supportive, loving atmosphere, regardless of what was happening.

One evening we evacuated to Samantha's parents house because a hurricane was coming. It was frightening, and it was the first time I'd ever seen devastation of that magnitude caused by a storm up close. However, when I looked around at Samantha's family, they were embracing and encouraging one another, assured they would make it through because they were together.

I found shelter with them, which helped with the transition when I moved into Dad and Samantha's house. Their acceptance gave me strength and courage to face the challenges ahead.

I had my first sexual relationship with a girl from school during that year, which was my senior year of high school. Being the new kid in school and in town, I didn't have to worry about what people thought about me or what they knew about my family.

Jan was beautiful, which was how I'd been taught to judge people. She had everything going for her – long sunshine kissed hair, blue eyes, and a beautiful figure. Aesthetically, she was perfect because of what she brought to the world with her physical appearance.

What she brought to the relationship, however, was an unhealthy need to manipulate and control. She thought nothing of throwing her drink in my face or telling me how pathetic I was because of a decision I had made. She was abusive and made unrealistic demands that made me constantly wonder if I was good enough for her.

As our relationship became more abusive, I fell deeper into the role of submission. She thought nothing of punching me in the head or slapping me. Though I realized this wasn't the kind of activity I saw in Samantha's parents' home, I didn't seem to be able to do anything about it. I didn't feel worthy of having someone love me for me.

That summer, Dad and Samantha invited us to take a vacation with them. I was nervous because she always treated me horribly in front of them, doing whatever she could to humiliate me. She surprised me, however, by saying I should go alone and spend some time with them.

I jumped at the chance to go with them to their condo in Destin, and enjoyed the first day on the beach and dinner cooked on the grill. The next day I began to feel unusually anxious. I felt I needed to get back to Jan. I guess I had not become accustomed to being treated properly. It was uncomfortable for me to feel peace and not feel anxious all of the time. Dad and Samantha were surprised but said okay when I told them I was going back and would pick up my things at their house.

It was a two-hour drive, and as I pulled back into Dad's driveway, I saw that Jan's car was there. I quietly pulled up because curiosity had gotten the best of me. I thought it was really odd that she'd be there with no one else at home. I got out of my car and instead of slamming my car door I pushed it as close as I could get it and then put pressure up against it until I heard the latch click. I softly walked across the driveway and up to the front door. I sneaked inside and noticed my bedroom door was closed, and some things in the living room were out of place. There was a pair of men's shoes that I didn't recognize as well as a baseball hat with an A on it for the Angel's baseball team lying on the coffee table.

I slowly opened the bedroom door, and saw her and another guy lying naked on my bed. I quickly and quietly shut the door and walked back out to my car. Dad and Samantha asked me to bring home one of their coolers since I wasn't going to be at the condo any longer and it would give them more room.

I quietly lifted my trunk, picked up the cooler, and walked on tiptoe back through the front to my bedroom door. I slowly turned the door knob and peaked through the crack. They were both lying there sleeping naked. I reached down and grabbed the cooler and gingerly walked across the carpet to the foot of the bed, I lifted the cooler lid and threw the entire cooler of cold water all over her and her companion.

What happened next looked like it came from a bad sitcom, but it was hilarious.

They both jumped out of bed, running around trying to find their clothes and get dressed to get away. I stood there furious but quiet. I then yelled, "get your shit and get out!" I felt as liberated as I did the day I told

Pop he would never abuse me again. As she walked by me, my girlfriend said, "You didn't have to do that."

I gave her a mean smile and said, "If you're going to act like a bitch in heat, then I'm going to treat you like one."

Once the emotions and the theatrics were past, the realization of what I had done began to sink in. I had been replaced, and she didn't have enough respect for me to just tell me in a simple conversation. It turned out the guy was her old boyfriend and they couldn't go to his house because he was twenty two and still lived at home, and so did she. She chose to bring him to my parent's house because she knew we were out of town.

The reality was I had never treated myself with the respect I deserved. As long as I felt unworthy, I would be treated as someone unworthy and this was the first realization I had of this treatment.

I also realized that the kind of relationship I had with Jan was nothing like what I'd seen with Samantha's family. There was no love, no understanding, no real appreciation that one person should have for another.

In retrospect, that breakup was the best thing that could have happened. I shouldn't have been in a relationship for many reasons. I had no idea who I was so I had nothing of value to bring to a relationship. I also had no concept of what a healthy relationship between two people really felt like.

I knew what I wanted to achieve because I'd witnessed it with Samantha's family and the love they displayed for one another. What I didn't know was how to find that kind of unconditional, supportive, and healthy place.

I decided I needed a better understanding of myself and to find out why I wasn't reaching my goals emotionally even though I had seen several therapists. I knew at this point what I wanted to study in college. I wanted a better, deeper understanding of psychology. I needed a better grasp of what made me who I was and a better understanding of the events that had taken place in my life.

I still feel like an outsider with Samantha's family only because I keep myself at a distance to be sure I do nothing wrong. I would never want anything to tarnish what I have with them.

CHAPTER 11

GROWING UP

Ihad just started my freshman year in college when Dad and Samantha finished renovating our house they had purchased on the river. From the kitchen you could see the dining room. The floor in the kitchen was made of the same beautiful split brick that was in her mother's house. The remodeling job was stunning and I was always surprised at how Samantha was able to visualize how beautiful the kitchen would be through all of the construction chaos. She constantly had some scented candle or oil burning to keep the house smelling pleasant instead of like construction materials. This particular night she had some jasmine candles burning on the counter top. While I was standing on the step I could see Dad and Samantha whispering by the kitchen sink. I heard her say, "Well, if you feel that way then we have to tell him." Dad turned, looked at me and then started walking in my direction. Samantha stayed by the sink with her arms crossed watching as Dad moved closer to me. It was a very awkward silence between the three of us. I could tell that he was uncomfortable about something and, based on her body language, it was obvious she didn't agree with what he was going to say. I was taller than he was because of the height difference from the step to the kitchen floor. He held his head down and with one sudden movement as if to say, get it over with, he looked at me and said, "Son, we have been talking it over and we think you should consider a trade or a career where you could be trained on the skills that you need to be

159

successful. I was thinking maybe a hair dresser or a flight attendant. I just don't believe you are intelligent enough to complete college." I was ashamed and so embarrassed that this was their opinion of me.

I know my grades aren't perfect but why would they think this about me? I study really hard and I can't imagine why they feel that I am not capable of completing college.

I needed to respond without letting him know how offended I was because I didn't want him to think he had hurt my feelings. I looked at him and with determination in my voice I replied, "I appreciate you both being concerned about me but based off of my first quarter grades, I think I am doing very well in school. My lowest grade is a C and the rest are A's so I am not sure why you would feel this way."

Dad turned and looked at Samantha as if to non-verbally say, now what, and she continued where he left off, "Grant, it is not that we don't think you can't do it we were just thinking you might do better by learning a trade. I know school is hard for you and we just wanted to give you this as an option. If you think you can handle it then I guess we were mistaken. We just don't know if you will be able to handle the classes as they get harder." I was trying to understand where they were coming from but I was still perplexed. Feeling vulnerable and mortified I crossed my arms and slowly sat on the step. I held my head down and fixed my eyes on the kitchen floor. I wanted to become invisible. I didn't know what to say because every bit of confidence I had gained my first semester of school by making good grades was just shattered.

I didn't even look up, I wanted to disappear and not have them notice I was no longer sitting there but I knew that would be impossible. Without lifting my head I said, "Do you mind if I go to my room for a little while? I know you just finished cooking dinner but I'm really not very hungry." Without really giving them the opportunity to answer I stood up and started walking towards my room. I was trying to hold back the tears as I walked away and could hear Samantha behind me saying "We didn't mean to hurt your feelings; we were just hoping you could understand where we were coming from. Please don't be upset." I was not upset but more in shock. They may have been of the opinion that I was not smart enough to go to college but I was not emotionless. Hearing them say that caused me to close up all of the doorways I had worked so hard to open.

I tried to and understand what I had done to give them that perception of me? I tried to be objective about what they were saying but I just couldn't reconcile it in my mind. I was hurt beyond words.

I don't want to be a flight attendant or cut hair for a living. If I study hard enough I know I can do it regardless of what they think of me.

With that thought, I worked as hard as I could and studied every day to keep ahead of the rest of the class. I realized I needed to finish up the quarter at the University of South Alabama and go back to Panama City and be with people who understood me.

Two days after the quarter had ended I moved. I was not going to let their opinion of my intelligence get the best of me so I began taking basic college classes at the local junior college. The first few classes I took were very easy classes. One was Music Appreciation and the other one was College Algebra. I made A's in both of them and was on an adrenaline rush from doing so well and proving to myself I was smart enough. I determined it was time to register for a class that was unfamiliar to me. I decided this way I would truly be able to verify if my intelligence was something lacking for college. I began going through the course catalog looking at all of the classes that were new to me. It was daunting at first because so many of the classes I believed were very hard. I read about Trigonometry and then Chemistry, neither of which seemed interesting. Finally I got to a course called General Psychology. It was a class to study the general field of psychology and was designed to provide an understanding of human behavior by studying the adaptation of the individual to his physical and social environment. I thought to myself, an understanding of human behavior, could this course really help me understand what it is that has happened to me and why it happened? I then started wondering, did I emotionally adapt to my physical and social environment all of these years. Is the abuse that I sustained something that will never go away? Is it something that will be with me forever?

I became intrigued with the idea of the class and couldn't stop fantasizing about the insight it might provide me on my own family. I felt it would be better than having my own therapist. I hoped by taking this course it would help me better understand why I am the way I am and why things happened to me the way that they did. When I saw the junior college was offering psychology classes for the semester, I immediately enrolled.

I was mesmerized by what I was learning. The one thing that impacted me the most was the understanding of "comfort zones." The more I learned the more I thought about my life. Comfort zones are not about what is healthy, but what is comfortable for you personally. In looking back at my relationships, I realized that I had sought out people who would humiliate me and discard me just as people had done when I was a child.

I continued to reflect as I was able to identify relationships in my life. I contemplated; *I dwell in being the victim and then look for a similar type of relationship again to continue the cycle. This is what I identify as comfortable because I am use to being treated in this way. When people treat me well, I become scared and feel unworthy of positive treatment. The reality is that I am worthy of it but I have never been exposed to it before which makes it horribly uncomfortable.*

I felt like someone had finally given me the secret to life. I continued on; All this time, I thought that comfort zones were a practical place to be, simply taking the expression at face value. The more I learned the more I realized that comfort zones can be healthy or unhealthy based on experiences. Some people are comfortable with chaos around them and others are comfortable having healthy lives and creating boundaries with others.

Not only was I able to understand this course, I was not able to turn the pages fast enough. I would go home after class and read the book for pleasure at night because I was just enamored by the subject. I then started to understand so many things about myself. I realized that people that are abused do not understand what it means to be healthy and often times that is why the cycles of abuse continue in families. The person committing the abuse is perpetuating the behaviors that they know and don't believe there is a reason to change because they have always done it that way and the victim doesn't know a different life either.

I immediately thought about Evelyn. All of these years she claimed to not to have been abused but her behavior indicates the contrary. Many times you hear of people in violent domestic situations, such as my sister, where the person being abused repeatedly returns to the abuser, which is what she did. They do this because that is where they think they function best; it is familiar. That setting is the only place they know how to survive. When they are put in a peaceful, safe environment, it is more than they can handle. The words "comfort zone" imply that it is a comfortable place. For me, it needs to be taken a step further and clarified whether it is a healthy place for all involved.

With this knowledge, I continued assessing my life and realized that I had sought out unhealthy relationships because of what I had experienced living with my family. I don't think I would have come to this realization without the two years I'd spent with Dad and Samantha, being exposed to healthy, happy relationships.

I didn't even know I was unhealthy. I just thought that everyone had family dynamics like mine. I was unconsciously convinced that the bad situations in the past were all I deserved. The side effect was that I was creating a present that was completely dysfunctional.

For the first time, I was clearly seeing the episodes of my past and the impact they had on my life as an adult.

With every class, I sat quietly in the corner and listened intently to the instructor. When we stopped for the day, I wanted to stand up and yell, "You can't stop there."

Once I completed that class I realized what some of the therapist I had seen had been trying to tell me. I was just not educated enough to comprehend. I became more determined than ever to understand who I was and what I needed to do to be emotionally strong. I desperately wanted to learn how to develop safe comfort zones so I could build a healthy, new life.

During that semester I started exercising building boundaries. I would go out with my friends and if I was not having a good time then I would let them know and leave. This was a huge step for me because in the past I would worry more about them being mad at me for leaving than my own enjoyment and stay to satisfy their needs. I also stopped over-committing to people. I had previously created a pattern of making plans with multiple people for the same night because I couldn't tell them no. I didn't want anyone's feelings to get hurt or have them abhor me.

I would spend the day prior to the overbooked night stressing over what to do, praying that one of them would call and cancel. I didn't have enough self esteem to say no and I desperately wanted to be wanted. I would end up not showing and then beg for forgiveness. This was the chaos I grew up in and I knew I had to continue to change this behavior. It was unfair to me and to the people in my life.

That same semester I met someone who would turn out to be one of the dearest friends I would ever have because they respected me and the fact that I set boundaries for myself.

I went to dinner with my friend Margaret, who is a truly beautiful woman. Margaret was tall with a body of a swimsuit cover model. Her hair is flaxen with a hint of strawberry around her temples. Her personality was infectious and her loyalty to our friendship was unmatched by anyone. We were just friends and every time we would go anywhere men would drool all over her ignoring my presence.

One night at dinner, our waiter for the evening, a guy named John, seemed at first to be no different. He was engaging and funny, telling us about being new to Panama City and asking if we knew the fun places to hang out. He gave us both the same amount of attention, and I was surprised because usually if their eyes connected with mine it was only because it was time for the tip.

I couldn't tell if he was hitting on Margaret or genuinely being nice. She had a real presence and exuded confidence. This was probably the result of her beauty and being an only child with doting and loving parents who worshipped her and gave her everything she'd ever wanted.

We had finished our meal and Margaret was checking her lipstick when John came back over and asked what every guy did right before asking her out, "So, how long have the two of you been together." We laughed and responded, "People ask us that all of the time because we are together a lot, but we are just very good friends. More like brother and sister than anything." The next question was not unexpected. I almost wanted to do a countdown one, two, three and here it is. Instead it was not the typical groveling invite, "Oh, well with that said, would you two like to go to Shipwreck Island with me tomorrow?" I was surprised for a moment because he had asked us both.

Margaret and I were both startled at his boldness, "Sure, it sounds like fun," Margaret responded clicking her makeup bag shut as she put it back into her purse.

He was being really nice, but I knew it was likely he was hoping I would cancel so he could be alone with her. He looked at the both of us as we stood up from the table and looked right into my eyes and said, "Great I will call you around ten o'clock in the morning."

As we headed for the door, I looked at her and said, "Well, it looks like you have yourself a date."

She paused in her tracks and took in a deep breath, "I hate to tell you this," she said. "But I can't make it tomorrow. I already have plans, and I'm not going to cancel them. It would be the second time I've had to do it, and I'm not going to do that to my dad." I was upset because she had led him on and he really seemed to be a nice guy.

I replied, "Well, you need to go back in there and tell him that we can't make it." Looking at me with her bright blue eyes she rebutted, "I can't do that to him, he was so nice. Why don't the two of you go? It will be fun! When he calls you tomorrow just tell him I can't make it; that something came up." I was trying to decide if this was a comfort zone issue or just a friend making bad commitments and dumping them on me.

We started walking again towards the car and I attempted to practice what I had learned in Psychology class. I wanted to better understand why she did this so as she reached for my hand, as she always did, I looked at her and asked, "Why didn't you tell John that you had plans when he invited us to go?" She put her head on my shoulder and grabbed my hand with both of hers, "I didn't remember until we got to the door. Don't worry I am sure you will both have fun."

The next morning I woke up early and went for a run so I would not look fat in my swim trunks just in case he didn't decide to cancel. I was six feet one inch and weighed one hundred and sixty pounds but still had a horrible body image. I came back and jumped in the shower. As I was drying off. I thought I heard the phone ring; I looked at the clock as I ran to answer it. It was already ten o'clock. I reached for the talk button and was incredibly nervous but I had no idea why. It was just a guy from the restaurant, so what's the big deal, I thought to myself.

I grabbed the phone and answered, "Hello?" I stopped thinking that maybe it was him calling to cancel and this way I wouldn't have to break the news to him that Margaret would not be able to go.

"Hey Grant, how are you? This is John. I am calling to see if you were ready to go." He sounded very excited about going to Shipwreck Island but I knew as soon as I broke the news to him, I would have the rest of the day to myself.

Trying not to act indifferent, I gave the news to him quick and painless, "I am sorry to tell you but Margaret had to cancel. She forgot she had previous plans with her Dad. She said for you to give her a call later and she would be happy to plan something with you." Knowing he would undoubtedly cancel, I flipped on the Television to listen to the morning talk shows.

I had plopped down on the couch when he said, "No problem, I am glad she is able to spend time with her Dad. I am still up for going if you're still interested." I was surprised and not really sure how to respond. I wasn't sure if I had heard him correctly so I clarified. "You still want to go?" I asked inquisitively.

"I sure do, I have wanted to go there since I moved to Panama City, but I don't want to go by myself." I was caught off guard. Then I thought about how I was working on identifying my comfort zones and realized this would be a good time to test them and maybe make a new friend in the process. Either way I was not really risking much.

"Sure, I am happy to go. It has been a while since I've gone and it sounds like a lot of fun. Did you still want to come and pick me up or do you want to meet me there?" I was proud of myself for taking control of the conversation and diving right into the conditions of transportation.

"I'll come and pick you up. Let me jump in the shower and I should be there in about thirty minutes." I was thrilled; I was exercising what I had learned in class and venturing out into new areas.

"Great, I will see you then!" I said enthusiastically.

It was exactly thirty minutes from the time I hung up the phone until I heard the knock on the door. That's impressive; he showed up right on time, I thought to myself. His punctuality alone made me comfortable because it showed he followed through on his commitments.

I jumped up and turned off the television that I had been listening to as background noise and grabbed my beach towel. I passed by the kitchen bar, picked up my sunglasses, threw them on my head and quickly headed toward the door.

As I greeted him, I looked over his shoulder and noticed an older model red Camero and instantly became apprehensive. Most of the guys that I knew that drove cars like that were drug smoking rednecks and it wasn't anything personal but I just didn't get into that scene. I paused and looked at him while he leaned up against the side of the door frame. *Oh, great,* I thought, *Margaret has attracted this man's man and I'm going to have to spend the day telling him how great she is and answering a ton of questions about her.* I had to remind myself, *this is to learn how to create boundaries based on what you are identifying as your comfort zone so don't worry about it. Tell him you don't want to talk about her all day and if he is alright with it then go and have fun.*

I looked right at him and abruptly dictated, "I am not going to spend the entire day telling you about Margaret. If that is what you hope to accomplish today then go ahead and let me know so I can answer your questions now and not waste your time or mine." It sounded much better in my head and as the words were crossing my lips it felt horrible. I think I could have delivered the message better, but at the same time it felt liberating.

"No problem, we don't have to mention her at all today if you don't want." He was casual and almost looked relieved when I told him. I didn't want to let my guard down so I continued in the same tone trying to show my independence. "Well, as long as we're clear." I turned to shut and lock the door and squinted my eyes thinking to myself, oh my gosh, I don't think I could have been any more rude but I don't want to lose this assertive side I am trying to develop.

I slung my beach towel over my shoulder, pulled the sunglasses that were resting on top of my head down over my eyes and walked out into the sun. I took in a deep breath and could smell the ocean. "I loved the smell of the beach this early in the day", I mumbled under my breath not wanting to sound like a dork.

John walked in front of me and made it to the car first. He opened his car door and the serenity of the morning was suddenly interrupted by a loud squeak. It was so loud that it startled me at first and I immediately stopped in my steps. It was coming from his car door and when he pulled the door to shut you could hear the solid thud it made when it connected with the frame of the car. It was undoubtedly a car that would withstand any kind of an accident. Once I regained my stride again I quickly reached the passengers car door, I looked in the open window, and John leaned over and said, "Hey, are you ready to have some fun?"

Surprised by his greeting, I got into the stifling car. The heat took my breath away at first. I was surprised that it was so hot this early in the morning. His car did not have air conditioning, and when I sat down on the red vinyl seats I could feel the heat start to singe the back of my legs. I quickly jerked my legs up so only the material from my shorts was touching. I pulled my towel off of my shoulder and shoved it under my legs. I was sweating instantly, but I replied, "Yes, I'm ready for a great day." The smell of the car reminded me of the old cars Pop use to work on. A bit of oil, mixed with age. "What year is your car," I asked him, trying to determine if he would be able to find replacement parts for the door that sounded like it was about to fall off.

"It's a seventy six and I worked for months so I could afford it. I love this car but it is a bit old." I couldn't quite identify what I was feeling but as he started to explain to me how hard he had worked for the car, I started to really appreciate its beauty. It was immaculate on the inside, the seats were in perfect condition and it was spotless. You could see the pride he had for this car everywhere.

Once we got moving, there was a great breeze, and the smell of the car had been replaced by the smell of the morning air. I closed my eyes and stuck my head out of the window a bit to feel the gentle stream of wind softly caress my hair and face. Realizing that I needed to establish a dialog, I looked at him and asked, "So where are you from again?" He smiled and said, "A small town outside of Joplin called Seneca, Missouri. I have three brothers and one sister and they all still live there. I couldn't stand living in such a small town so I looked at a map and picked a place to move and that is how I wound up here in Panama City." I was surprised and continued with the questioning, "You're telling me that you just looked at a map, saw a spot that looked interesting, packed up your things, and left? What did your family say?" At this point he was smiling ear to ear, I was listening attentively because I admired his courage to do something so spontaneous.

He continued, "I am the youngest of all of my siblings. I have three brothers that are twenty one, nine and six years older than me and my sister is eight years older. They are already established in their lives so they didn't really have too much to say."

I was engaged by his story so I continued, "Oh, my gosh, your oldest brother is almost my mom's age. If you are the baby of the family then how old are you?" He had a moustache and looked much older than me so I was guessing his age to be around twenty three. He looked at me boastfully and blurted, "How old do you think I am?" I didn't want him to feel uncomfortable so I thought I would guess a number that was lower than what I thought. I reactively said, "I would think you are at least twenty one." He turned and looked at me as if I had just told him he was as old as dirt and said, "Well, I am nineteen." Afraid I had stepped on his pride, I started to back track. "I can see that, it is just that your moustache makes you look a bit older."

With a smirk on his face he began to question my age, "So, how old are you?" Wanting to make up for embarrassing myself I said, "I am as young as you are."

He smiled and started to laugh and talk, "When is your birthday?" Smiling back I responded, "September fourth, why when is yours?" Appearing as if he had just won a scratch off lottery ticket he yelled, "HAH! You are older than me by a month and sixteen days. My birthday is October twentieth."

Realizing I had hurt his ego a bit by guessing he was older I continued along with this sparring correspondence and changed my voice to sound like an old man. "Well then Sonny, you might have to help me around the park today when we get there."

We both loudly burst out in laughter. Most of it was because we were really having a good time but some of it was still nervousness.

The time had passed by so quickly that when I looked from him to the front windshield, we were already pulling into the parking lot. I was a little amazed that he never mentioned Margaret during the trip.

When I got out of the car I could hear the water rides in the background and the burning scent of chlorine was potent. We approached the admission gate to see a young blonde girl selling tickets. I reached in my pocket to pull out my money and John put his hand out motioning for me to keep my money.

"I'll get it; I was the one that invited you so I don't expect you to pay." I was surprised by his generosity and started to get a bit fearful that it was a big joke.

I pulled my hand out of my pocket, smiled and with gratitude said, "Wow, I didn't expect that. Thank you so very much." He turned, smiled and shrugged his shoulders as if to say, "No big deal."

As we walked through the turn wheel that counted our entrance into the park, I began to tell him about my Psychology class and how much I was enjoying college. Concerned I was talking too much about school; I stopped talking and asked, "Do you go to school?" With an almost rehearsed answer as if he had been asked the question a million times he said, "I hope to go one day but I am not sure about it yet. It is really expensive." I was sad for a second and then continued, "You can get student loans to pay for it, and you don't have to pay anything back until you are done taking classes or when you graduate." Consolingly he whispered, "I know but I just don't know if college is for someone like me."

I finally got the message and ended the conversation. I looked around at all of the people yelling and screaming as they slid down water slides and ran from one ride to the other. Just like the kids around us, John looked at me enthusiastically, "Come on let's go." Off we went to try and recapture some of our childhood.

We stayed at the park all day and were starving as we left that evening. We decided to continue the day with dinner, and I thought nothing about it because we were having such a great time together. He suggested we go by my house so I could shower and change and then head to his place so he could do the same. My house was closer to the park, so it just made sense to go there first.

When we got there, Mom was home, and I introduced her to John. I told her about our dinner plans and headed off to get into the shower while she and John got acquainted. I couldn't hear what they were saying but I was fearful that she would tell him things about me that were not true or exaggerate something that I would regret later. She would often fictionalize the truth and I would be asked about it later and feel uncomfortable for not supporting what she had said. Once, she had told one of my friends that she was a body builder when she was younger. I was standing there and it was the first time in my thirteen years I had ever heard that before. Later on they questioned me about it and my only response was, "if that is what she says then I guess it is true."

The reality was, she was trying to somehow justify the fact that she was overweight by telling people how thin she use to be and how beautiful she use to be. The reality was she was still beautiful but didn't have enough self-esteem to be confident. I ran into my bedroom to pick out my clothes. I often struggle the most when trying to decide on what to wear because I wanted people to like me. I believed that if the shirt was not likable by others then I was not likeable. I know that it made no sense but if I didn't look good then I always feared others would view me as unworthy somehow. If my clothes looked cheap then I must be less in the eyes of others.

After about twenty minutes I took the clothes I had chosen into the bathroom and rushed through my shower so that I could stop the conversation he and Mom were having. I pulled on my clothes and I could feel them sticking to my body where I had missed places when I dried off. I went running out of the bathroom saying loudly, "Ok, I am almost finished just give me a few more minutes," hoping to interrupt. I threw on my shoes and barreled around the corner into the kitchen where John had been talking with her while sitting on one of the bar stools. I took over the conversation immediately, "I'm ready when you are." Mom looked at me and said "Well, that was fast." I didn't want her to know the real reason why so I replied, "I am starving and he still has to get ready." I snatched my wallet and keys from the counter and headed for the door while saying, "I will see you later." Closing the door without hearing her response, John looked at me with surprise and said, "She sure is a talker." Apparently they talked nonstop while I got ready. "Well, whatever she said that seems impossible to believe, trust yourself." I laughed and headed towards his car and back to his house so he could get ready.

As we turned onto the street where he lived I was really impressed. He lived in an attractive townhouse. I was surprised he was as young as me and able to be so independent.

We walked up to the door and I couldn't help but wonder what was behind it. As he opened the door I was taken aback. Trying not to act alarmed, I looked around in amazement. The stairwell was directly to the left. To the right was a huge room that included a living room and dining room combined. It was beautiful. The couch was right under the windows along the same wall as the front door. It was white, and looked like a huge cloud. He had an entertainment center that was up against the wall of the stair case and included a television, VCR and a stereo system. Past the living room was a glass-top dinette that incorporated four black chairs with mauve cushions. Behind the dining room table was a Nagel print of a woman with short hair wearing mirrored sunglasses. It was a black and white drawing with splashes of purple on her lips and the fabric that she had draped just past her shoulders.

He stopped me as my eyes darted around the room, "I am going to go upstairs and get dressed, it should take about ten minutes." I was embarrassed because I knew it took me twice that long just to pick out something to wear, "No problem," I responded, "I'll just sit here and wait." As I reached out to touch the couch I couldn't get over how amazingly soft it was. I couldn't figure out what the fabric was but it had to be some type of a micro fiber or suede. He turned and I could hear his thumps as he ran up every step and then once he reached the top it stopped and I heard his door close.

While he got ready, I surveyed the downstairs area, getting more impressed because of his nice furnishings, a fully stocked kitchen, and the amazing colors he had painted on the walls. One wall was gray and the other one was a mauve color that matched the seats of the dinette. I looked out of his sliding glass doors and saw a very small nicely groomed back yard.

I was thinking to myself, *how does he afford all of this*, when I heard him coming back down the stairs. I don't even think it took all of ten minutes and I started back toward the couch. I didn't want him to think that I had been snooping around. As soon as I hit the cushion, he hit the bottom step. I looked up at him and was awestruck. I didn't know exactly what I was feeling, but I knew I had made an incredible connection. A few seconds later I was enveloped by the strong scent of his cologne. It was so powerful it was starting to burn my eyes a bit.

I didn't want to be rude so I asked, "What is that cologne you're wearing?" he proudly come back with, "It's a new cologne I have called Drakkar Noir. I just put it on so I hope it isn't too strong."

I didn't have the heart to tell him it was overpowering me so I just smiled and said, "No, not at all it just smells really good."

He opened the door, and I took a jaunty step outside, feeling I was doing a great job at making friends and setting boundaries.

We got in the car and I couldn't hold it in any longer, "Just curious, do you have any roommates?" I was hoping I had not crossed a line. The fact was that he is the only person I had known that didn't live with his parents.

"I do, I have two roommates, why do you ask?" It all started to come together and make sense. He obviously shared a place with them and that stuff was not all of his. "Oh, I was just curious because your place was so nice and well decorated." Knowing he was about to tell me that it was not his, he surprised me. "Thank you," he said with a tone that took ownership of the things in his house. I quickly turned my head, "you mean that all of the furniture in your house is yours? You bought all of those things?" He smiled and with pride responded "Yes, it is all mine. I have been working extra shifts to decorate the place. So, do you like it?" I didn't know what to say. I wanted to tell him how everything we have is only because Mom got it in the divorce and that most of it was about twenty years old. I didn't want him to judge me so I humbly answered, "Yes, it is nice. I think you have done a great job."

We agreed that we were both starving and craving pizza. We went to Pizza Hut and I devoured most everything on the salad bar and ate about five slices of pizza. We talked about life, people we had known growing up, and things that excited us. I was amazed he'd just picked a place on the map and moved there with no fear at all. "Yep, I just realized that where I was didn't work for me anymore and thought Panama City would be a better place. I looked at him and asked "Well, is it a better place?" With a long pause staring into my eyes he softly said, "Yes, much."

We finished dinner and went back over to his townhouse so I could meet his roommate. I was excited because if he was anything like John, then he too would make a great friend.

We walked in. I assumed my place on the couch while John went to look for his roommate. He ran upstairs screaming, "Steve, are you here? Hello." I could hear him knocking on his bedroom door. He returned from upstairs, "I guess he's out." and he came over and plopped down on the couch beside me. As he sat down, his arm went up on the back of couch, and I didn't think anything of it.

We continued to talk and I could tell that the tension between us had changed and become clumsy. I was still talking and he was giving me one or two word answers, unlike before. He suddenly looked at me and said, "Can I kiss you?"

I froze and said, "Why?"

"Because I think you're great."

I was totally confused, thinking he meant a kiss on the cheek and wondering if it was some kind of Missouri custom I knew nothing about. I didn't want him to feel awkward so I leaned forward and offered him my cheek.

Laughing, he said, "What are you doing?"

"I thought you wanted a kiss."

"I do, but not on your cheek, on your lips," he said quietly.

To say I was freaked out is a not an exaggeration. I was excited, nervous, and wanted to puke all at the same time. I didn't know what to do. I thought about my psychology class, but realized we hadn't talked about this at all.

I knew he wasn't gay because he lived in a very nice place and all I was told growing up is that gay people lived in trailer parks, smelled terrible, were drug users, and had sex only at parks and bathrooms. I didn't think he had exhibited signs of deviant behavior and he certainly didn't smell funky. I had seen no signs of drug abuse but I didn't even know what the signs were.

Confused beyond words I decided to use what I had learned about conflict resolution. I needed to clarify what was happening. I looked at him and said, "You know, I hear what you are saying, but I don't get why you are saying it."

"I think you are cute, and I just thought it would be a fun thing to do," he said like he was explaining something to a child. With that, I decided he must be exploring new things. I knew about that. We had studied it in class. We discussed the kiss a little more, "Are you talking full tongue action or just a peck on the cheek? I just want to be sure I meet your expectations if I do this." He leaned forward and said, "Let's just see what happens," and I decided to give it a try. As I approached his lips, I couldn't believe what I was doing. I was pretty certain I would burn in hell for the rest of my life for doing this based on the religious beliefs I had grown up with. Then our lips touched, and I felt butterflies' in my stomach. It felt amazing. There was no remorse, and, frankly, I wasn't sure I wanted to stop doing it. When we moved apart, he looked at me and said, "Are you okay?" I smiled and said, "Yes, I think I am."

That tentative kiss was the starting point of a wonderful new life that I never knew existed. John helped me learn about boundaries and how to establish them in a healthy way. He taught me how to be independent, set goals and he supported me unconditionally. He taught me that love is separate from sex because we loved one another as people and sex was not part of the equation at first. Because we were the same age, I was shocked he knew so much about relationships.

I continued going to school and became very intrigued with this new relationship. This was the first time I would sit and miss someone that I had just seen less than an hour prior. When I would see him again, I could feel my heart beat a million times an hour. I didn't understand it but I didn't want it to be different because it was the first time in my life that

I connected with someone that seemed to love me for all of my weirdness and hang-ups.

Six months after dating I moved into his beautiful townhome. A year or so later we decided to move to Orlando. Moving to a new place seemed like a good idea, because I was still trying to hide my relationship with John from my friends and family.

The first week we were there I registered for school at the University of Central Florida and got a full-time and part-time job. John and I both waited tables and I washed clothes at Walt Disney World. It was great money, and I needed a lot of it so I could afford to go to school and graduate without being ridiculously in debt.

I decided to make the most of my education so that I would get out of it what I needed to better understand my life. When I found classes I needed to take, I made appointments with all of the professors to get an expectation of the class and the professor. I didn't want to spend my money on them and not learn anything and I was not looking for a class that would give me an easy "A".

There were several professors that I passed on because they thought it was ridiculous that I would interview them before taking their class. That was a red flag for me right away.

There were three classes I knew I needed to take immediately to better understand what was happening in my life. While others were in therapy, I was absorbed in my psychology classes, trying to learn as much as I could about my mental health. I didn't know if I were gay, straight, bisexual or just someone desperate to belong and be loved.

The first class was sexual behavior, which helped me understand there was nothing abnormal about being attracted to another man. They didn't all live in trailer parks, and the ones that I knew that did were wonderful, loving people. There was nothing wrong with living in a trailer or living in a mansion, as long as you were a good person.

I also learned the true definition of a sexual deviant, which helped me understand what Pop had done to me. It wasn't me that was the problem, it was his childhood that made him who he was and he never bothered to break the cycle. Instead he perpetuated it by abusing me. I discovered how to define sexual boundaries. This helped me realize Pop was a clearly-defined child molester and sexual predator.

Another class that fascinated me was the Psychology of Blacks. I was really missing having Nelly in my life, and being in this class helped me understand what she and I represented with our relationship. I learned about the history of racism, the beauty of the African-American culture, and how misunderstood Nelly was by my family because they subscribed to hateful racist beliefs. I despised them even more for this and began to wonder if Pop had ever raped her because of the fear she had shown around him.

The last class I took helped me to understand the choices Evelyn had made. Called "Women in Crime," it explained the criminal mind of a woman and the different elements that force women into those situations. This class also provided me with information about one of the most important aspects of psychology: the cycle of abuse.

As soon as we began studying this, I realized it was exactly what was happening in my life and in my family. Most importantly, it helped me understand why my sister had resorted to such drastic measures to get away from her abusive husband. Desperate times call for desperate measures is not just an old adage. She had gotten stuck in this cycle and while she would tell everyone that nothing had happened to her, she exhibited, more than anyone else, the signs of being abused as a child. She would be friends with anyone that gave her attention, regardless of their character. She never stood up for herself and allowed people to take advantage of her because she had no sense of self-worth.

John and I had clearly defined healthy boundaries and unconditional guidelines. I was feeling better about my financial situation because I was making enough money to have a car, pay for my schooling, my rent, and other necessities. I was happy and I loved my life.

John and I had been together for seven years when something I never thought would happen, did. One night I was waiting up for him to come home. Every hour I would look at the clock, and then every thirty minutes which quickly became every minute. It was three in the morning when I was calling hospitals in the area, police stations, the sheriff's office and the highway patrol. It is hard to explain, but when you are as close as we were I could feel that something terrible had happened. I had dialed until five o'clock in the morning with no luck finding him anywhere. Finally, I heard the door knob turn. I jumped up and ran towards the door and as I approached, in walked John. I was flooded with emotions. I was so happy to see him and so mad that he had not called me. As, I went to hug him I could see that there was shame all over his face. "What happened? Where have you been? Why didn't you call?" I was asking the questions so fast that he never had the opportunity to answer.

He couldn't look me in the eyes and I knew what had happened, "I'm sorry," he softly whispered before continuing. "The entire way home, I have been trying to decide how I was going to be able to tell you this. Last night I met another guy and I stayed over at his house."

I was confused at first because what he was saying did not make any sense, "What, you spent the night with who?" Still unable to look at me he responded, "I don't want to tell you who he is because you know him. He works with me and you have met him before." About that time it all started to sink in. It would have been easier had someone shot me in the heart instead of betraying me like he had just done. I could feel everything that I knew about my life changing with this conversation. Everything that I loved and cherished so much was no longer going to be.

My insides started to feel as if they were going to boil and tears clouded my sight. I looked at him and said, "What did I do? What did I do to make you want someone else?" Without even taking a breath he quietly said, "It wasn't you, it is me, I want different things in my life that I just don't think you can give me. I don't want to be tied down to someone right now." I appreciated his honesty but at that particular time I would have preferred a lie.

My heart break became rage within just a few seconds. He violated everything I had found security in, after all of our conversations about trust and respect. Outraged, I ran into the bedroom and started grabbing his clothes. I was pulling them out of the closet and throwing them onto the front lawn. I was being irrational. He patiently stood and watched. As I threw a pile, he would walk behind me and pick them up never saying a word, letting me get it all out. He knew me well. Finally, I collapsed onto the floor and started screaming. "How could you do this? How could you leave what we've built for seven years and throw it all away like this? You don't even want to try and work things out? You need to give me more than a speech about it being all you and not me."

He dropped down to the floor with me and said, "I know you want me to tell you it's you but it's honestly not. I've been feeling this way now for a few months and last night it just hit me that we just want different things." Furious that he would say something about his night I hatefully said, "Well, I guess what ever hit you last night you will keep on hitting." I jumped up and ran into the living room and started screaming. "Take your shit, take it all, and get the hell out of here." I picked up a chair from the same dinette that he had when we met and started throwing them out onto the front yard. Next out onto the lawn was his couch and then the coffee table. The adrenaline was so intense I could have picked up a refrigerator and thrown it out.

He snatched up his car keys and stormed out the door. If he was trying to tell me anything I had no idea what it was because I had become belligerent with my words and behavior. Once everything, including the silverware, had been thrown out into the yard, I sat down in the middle of the empty room and began to weep. John was everything I had known since being in Orlando. I couldn't afford where I was living without him and I had no place to go because I didn't know anyone that well. More than that, I didn't trust anyone like I trusted, or thought I trusted him.

A few minutes later the neighbor that lived behind us came and knocked on the door. With the first thud of his knuckle the door started to creep open and he saw me sitting on the floor crying. "What's wrong?" he asked, "I heard some yelling and banging and wanted to come and check on you guys. I was quick to respond, "After being together for seven years John just told me that he is no longer interested in continuing our relationship. I have nowhere to go, I don't know anyone and I don't know what to do." He cautiously knelt down and placed his arm around my shoulders and I fell into his body.

He stroked my hair as I drenched his shirt with my tears. His name was Mark Black. He was from Chicago and probably one of the nicest people I had met during my time in Orlando. He was about five feet eight inches, twenty eight years old and worked for one of the big companies' in town. He was college educated and had recently broken up with his partner. He looked at me and suggested, "You know I have an extra bedroom now and you are more than welcome to stay with me if you would like until you get on your feet." Of all the people to say this to me, I couldn't believe it was him. I admired him so much because of he was living the life I felt I wanted; being successful, working for a company Monday through Friday with weekends off and financially secure.

I pulled my head away from him and looked up into his green eyes and said, "Are you sure you don't mind?" By this point I was positive snot was likely running down my face but it didn't matter to me. I just wanted to get out of there and find a place where I did not feel so vulnerable. Without hesitation he looked at me and said, "Of course I am sure. We can talk about how long you want to stay later. Let me help you grab some things and bring them on back." He helped me up and I packed a few necessities and we went back to his apartment.

About a week later I had moved all of my things into Mark's apartment. Living with him was wonderful. For the first time in my life I was living on my own but I had Mark as my training wheels just in case I fell over.

One day I was sitting on his couch while he cooked dinner. I was telling him about a party that I was invited to but didn't really want to go. He looked at me and said "What's the worst thing that could happen?" I stopped mid thought and said, "Wow! That is the same thing Nelly use to tell me. I had forgotten about how powerful those words are. I think I need to remind myself of these words more often." He looked at me puzzled and asked, "Who is Nelly?" Smiling, I said, "She is the greatest human being that has ever graced this earth. She was like a mother to me growing up and I have not thought about her is several years. I have been too caught up with me to think about her, I guess. She kept me safe when I was younger."

Being respectful as he always was he didn't press for any more details and gently said, "She sounds like an awesome lady and you were lucky to have her in your life." With a smirk on my face I thought, *you have no idea.*

A month after living with Mark, John showed up and knocked on the door. He began to babble about how he had made a terrible mistake and that he wanted to take it all back. I realized that I was starting to get over the entire situation and that I really loved living with Mark and doing my own thing. I flatly said, "I am sorry that things didn't work out with you and that other guy but I am really happy. I think you are right, it wasn't me it was you." I smiled as I shut the door. By the time he got back to his apartment he called me. "I just want you to know I am sorry." I was hurt by what happened but I think it was the best thing for me. I loved him as a friend but didn't want anyone in my life as a partner any longer and said, "I understand and I do miss you but I think it is best we stay just as friends. Can you be open to that?" With a smile in his tone, I heard him get choked up and say, "Yes, for now that will be great."

When we realized our relationship was getting back to the level of just friendship, we decided that we did in fact love each other, but more like brothers.

CHAPTER 12

TRUST ME.....

I had finally found an apartment and moved out of Mark's place about three months after moving in. Now that I was living in an apartment alone, I was completely dependent on myself for the first time. During this time, I had some very unconventional jobs to help cover my expenses. I found I thoroughly enjoyed living alone, being able to make my decisions without having to get input from others. I made some good ones and some bad ones, but they were all good life lessons for me.

It was the same way with friends. Some were better than others, but with my newly learned skills of creating safe boundaries that both Mark and John had taught me, I was focused on achievement. I knew I wanted an emotionally happy and prosperous life without worrying about anyone but myself. I was making great strides at work and enjoyed being a part of the Human Resources Department, finally working Monday through Friday. I had coworkers who recognized my abilities and coached me and helped me advance in ways I never thought possible.

Some of my coworkers tried to talk me out of getting my degree in psychology, but once they realized what passion I had for the subject, they acknowledged it was the right thing for me to do. I was frequently questioned about my choice of majors, and mostly people wanted to know what I'd be able to do in the workforce with a degree in psychology. I was always delighted by their confused faces when I responded, "Be healthy."

As my professional career in Human Resources began an upward trend, my financial resources began to decline. I realized I was going to have to make some sacrifices. I wanted to work with some of the best companies around, so I knew I needed to establish a solid resume since I couldn't afford an Ivy League education. This meant I needed to make some job changes to increase my responsibilities at work and possibly take a cut in pay. Waiting tables paid great, but it did not provide the career advancement I was seeking. I needed to continue my education while working toward career goals without getting myself deeply in debt with college loans.

One night, some friends begged me to go to a new club with them. I'd been avoiding the social scene, focusing all my energy on my jobs and school. I decided it might be a good time to take a break from responsibility, so I agreed to go along. I even volunteered to be the designated driver since I'm not a drinker and have no interest in the drug scene.

The club was remarkable, with people dancing on speakers and the dance floor down below them. The lights were chaotic and illuminating all over the place. As you walked down the long hallway entrance, on the right was a bar and across the dance floor was the second one. There was a sitting area that was decorated with couches, huge oversized velvet drapes and overstuffed chairs where people were sitting and chatting. I loved to dance and I could feel the vibration from the music, so I took off for the dance floor immediately. My friends and I were laughing and having a great time. A little later in the evening, still on the dance floor someone tapped me on the shoulder. I stopped and turned around to discover a very familiar looking lady. I couldn't remember where we'd met. She leaned towards my ear and loudly said, "Can you step to the side of the dance floor?" As soon as I heard her voice I recalled her name instantly, Cindy. She was the promotions director for another club in town. I had met her at a friend's house one night and she was telling me all of the dirt on the bartenders, dancers and drag queens.

She was a lady of few words so I panicked, wondering if I'd been dancing in an area reserved for something else, and this was the only way she could get me to move. As we approached the side of the dance floor, the music got louder. She grabbed me by my hand and led me to another area of the club that was out of conspicuous sight and somewhat quieter. It was a makeshift office behind a glass door that looked more like a prop than an actual door. In the room was a light and a desk with a chair behind it and that was it. It was very gangster-like and I expected her to have a pile of cocaine or money sitting on the desk with Guido or Vinny standing on each side of the door. As we stopped, I began apologizing. She stopped me in mid-sentence.

"I've been trying to find your phone number for more than a month," Cindy said.

I wasn't sure how to respond to that, so I blurted, "Why?"

"I have been offered the job as promotions director here," she said, "and I want you to be one of our dancers."

I thought she was joking because everyone knew I wasn't the party animal type at all. A night at a club was a rare treat for me. I began laughing and said, "I don't think that will fit my school schedule too well."

Unfazed by my words, she went on about the job, which included tips, a guarantee of five hundred dollars a week, and some travel. I didn't hear anything else after she mentioned how much it would pay because this seemed to be the answer to my prayer. It would allow me to do what I needed for school, work and give me a chance to pursue the career I wanted. This is not the type of job I was looking at for a resume builder but it would allow me the financial means to take the lower paying jobs that would help support my Human Resources career growth while still affording school.

Before she could finish her speech, I was ready to sign on the dotted line. When she said, "Will you do it?" I screamed, "Yes, I will do it."

"Are you serious?" she asked, studying my face.

"Of course I am," I said, keeping my face as serious as possible. Curious, I asked, "Why are you interested in me doing this out of all the possible people you could find who'd do it?"

"Well, you're nothing like all the other possibilities. You have a great head on your shoulders; you're a responsible person, and a face not everyone recognizes because you don't live here in the club every weekend."

I was ecstatic! I rejoined my friends on the dance floor. Feeling like I'd just won a major competition, I was hesitant to share my news with them because I knew they would judge me for agreeing to this, but I was focused on my future.

When it came time to go to work the next weekend, I was really nervous. I'd never done anything like this before and couldn't imagine getting paid for having so much fun. Cindy met me at the door. "Hey there I am so excited you made it."

Almost too scared to utter a word I looked at her and said, "Thanks, I am so freaking nervous," as I shook my hands at my sides to dry the sweat from my palms. "Come on in and I'll show you where to get changed," she said as the door closed behind me.

We walked through the club and the lights seemed to come alive as the music filled the room. I was looking around in awe at what the place looked like with so few people in it. The smell was the same, like smoke and dried liquor.

She led me up to a set of stairs that looked like they belonged to a fire escape. At the top was a landing, a door, and white drapery that surrounded the wall.

"This is where all of the dancers hang out and get ready before their sets." She yelled down to me as I looked up at her butt following her up the stairs.

From the top of the landing you could look over the entire club and see that it was previously a garage, which is how it got its name Club Firestone after the Firestone garage that use to be there. The dance floor was sunken and obviously where the mechanics went to change the oil for their cars. There was a bar on the upper level and one on the lower level by the dance floor. To the left of the lower bar was where the sitting area was located.

On the right side of the door were white sheet-looking curtains that created a big square tunnel around the ceiling of the dance floor but from there you could see that it was a cat walk that went around the dance floor with ladders that dropped down over each of the speakers. There were four speakers, one in each corner, and they were about ten feet high off of the dance floor and about two feet above the second level. To get onto the speakers you had to walk out on the cat walk, find the speaker you were assigned to, try to inconspicuously climb down the ladder and join the other dancer in mid rhythm. Then the dancer that was relieved could take an hour break, climb back up the ladder and then walk back to the third floor room to join all of the others there.

When she opened the door, I saw several people that I did not know. They all glared over their shoulders and some looked through the reflections of the mirrors at me. None of them spoke. I was clearly the new kid on the block.

Cindy looked down at my book bag and asked, "What it is in there? We don't encourage drug use back here." I started laughing as I opened my bag and told her, "I have my school books with me so I can study if I get any free time. Don't worry, I don't do drugs."

She smiled and said, "I definitely made a great decision when I hired you."

She took me to a corner of the dressing room where I could change. I had brought a pair of shorts and my favorite boots to make my dancing debut. I heard the music get louder and the crowd poured in the doors. Pulling all of the study material out of my book bag, I was ready to get to work when I looked around the dressing room at the other dancers.

Some were drinking and some were doing drugs, which really shocked me. *So much for not doing drugs up here,* I thought to myself.

Being there was surreal to me, I felt as if I didn't belong, but at the same time, I didn't feel threatened by anyone. They did their own thing and I was doing mine. We weren't really so different, they got high from the drugs and I was getting a high from the thought of making money. Seeing everyone's behavior also confirmed that I was in exactly the right place, sitting in the back corner studying, because that kind of life held absolutely no interest for me. I didn't judge them; it was just a different path, one that I was not willing to go down. I had enough issues with control and I didn't want substances, especially illegal ones, altering my path or state of mind. This job was a means to an end.

Cindy came back and asked "would you come with me for a minute?"

She could tell by my dazed and lost look that I was not sure what to do. "Sure, no problem," I got up, moved my books to the side and began walking toward her.

She grabbed my hand and leaned forward and whispered, "The other dancers are very aggressive and might try to steal your things, be smart about where you leave your stuff and don't trust anyone but Desiree. She will teach you what you need to know and take care of you." I had no idea who Desiree was. When we first walked in and I was looking around I had noticed dancers already out there and assumed she was one of them.

As we walked out, she told me, "Your set is about to begin, and I really want you to get the best speaker on the floor."

She pointed to the one closest to the second floor bar. I quickly realized why. It was the one that was most easily accessible by patrons. If you were going to the bar or coming to the dance floor you had to walk by it. Who got which speaker was very political and was as competitive as being the next person chosen for a promotion. Being in a prominent place meant more exposure to the guests, which also meant more money. As we walked out of the door, she pulled the sheer white curtain back and motioned for the girl dancing on the most desired speaker to join us.

That must be Desiree, I thought.

Desiree reached up and pulled on the ladder to climb up and meet us. We walked out on the cat walk and when she got to the top rung of the ladder I reached down and grabbed her hand. She flipped her hair back with one swift motion and let out a huge, "whew." She was incredibly beautiful like she was made by Mattel.

Cindy introduced us, "Desiree, this is Grant. He's the new guy I was telling you about that would be splitting sets with you." I was mesmerized by her because she looked so perfect. She was wearing a metallic silver bra top that matched her shorts and go-go boots.

"I stuck my hand out without taking my eyes off of hers, stuttering out the words, "Nice to, um, hey, I mean, what's going on." I was trying to be cool but instead sounded like an idiot. I didn't want her to get the impression that I was a dork, but I was afraid it was already too late.

Desiree looked me over and said with a sweet sexy voice that sounded like a cross between Demi Moore and Kathleen Turner, "It's great to meet you." Her eyes were sparkling from the glitter she had spread across her eye lids and her lips were full and perfectly colored with lipstick.

She continued, "I will be back in about an hour, so while I'm in the green room, I'll watch your stuff for you."

She looked over at Cindy and asked, "Do you mind showing me where he put his things? I want to make sure those vultures back there don't ruin his first night."

Cindy replied, "Of course, I'll walk you back." They turned to walk away and she did a quick sweep under the hem of her shorts to adjust them.

As she passed me, she slapped my ass and added, "Go out there and shake what yo' mama gave ya and have fun."

I loved her smile and her confidence. I looked back at Cindy and said, "So this is it, right?"

"It sure is. Are you okay?" I took a deep breath and I started my descent down to the speaker and said, "I guess. If I'm not, I will let you know when you get back."

She yelled and said, "Flirt like they are the hottest people you've ever seen."

I climbed down and was almost petrified when I started looking around. I could see people just staring at me and I was just starring back. I couldn't even hear the music because fear was starting to take over. I knew I had to do this so I could continue my education and I asked myself, *what's the worst thing that can happen?*

Once I began dancing on top of the speaker, people were gathering around to give me money and tips. I was shocked. All I was doing was dancing in a pair of shorts and these people were throwing money at me like I was a bartender serving free drinks for tips. I was so excited, and once the adrenaline kicked in, I did everything I could to get people's attention.

I would drop down onto the speaker and move my hips and pelvis around in an erotic motion simulating sexual movements and people would go wild. I lay on my back and let people rub their hands across my chest and they would drop money in my waistband, boots and on the speaker itself.

The time flew by and I had obviously danced about an hour because Desiree came out to relieve me. As she got closer and began to climb down, I reached up to help being the chivalrous persons that I am. When she stepped down, the people around us went crazy. Desiree asked if I'd mind dancing with her a few minutes to get the crowd ready for her dance, and I said sure.

I felt one of her legs go around my waist and the other one go around my neck. She tilted herself back until her head almost touched the floor and she rubbed her hands up and down her belly and across her chest. I could feel her body tremble and shake due to the tremendous physical control she was exuding to look this sexy. I really didn't know what to do but hang on for dear life and the entire time all I could think was *please don't fart in my face.*

I knew if she fell I'd go down right along with her because she had such a tight grip around me with her legs. As she continued to perform, people around us started screaming like crazy, and that seemed to do it for her. She was in incredible shape because her movements were so fluid like and smooth on the outside but I could feel how hard she was working to control her body. She used her abdominals and pulled herself back up and slowly slid herself down my body like I was a greased pole. She gave me a kiss and said, "Thanks, I'll see you in an hour" and smiled from ear to ear.

As I made my way back up the ladder and across the catwalk, I was shocked to see how many people were in the club. It was such an exciting place. Opening the door to the green room, I found people doing lines of cocaine, smoking pot, having sex and drinking. I lowered my head and made my way back to the corner where my books were and sat down. Just as she had promised, my books were there and things were well.

I began pulling money out of my boots and my shorts, finding everything from one dollar bills to a fifty dollar bills. During that first set, I had made more than two hundred and fifty dollars.

Oh, my God, I can't believe this!

It had been so easy. I put the money in my book bag and grabbed my books to try to begin studying but I could barely get the smile off of my face.

I loved what I was doing and by the end of that first weekend, I had made more than fifteen hundred dollars. I also had plenty of time to study and was ready for my exam on Monday.

I kept telling myself that it was the money that was making me feel so high, but I began to realize that it was the high from being treated like someone special that was doing it. All of it was superficial and I started hearing over and over again how gorgeous I was and what a beautiful body I had. *What a great ass* was always the most common comment. I started to realize that the longer I did this, the more I felt like a male hooker.

The reality was, everything they described was external. These people that were looking at me assumed I was someone that was willing to do anything for a dollar. None of them thought that I was a hard working, college educated person trying to help pay the bills.

I started to get treated as an object instead of a person. It was great for my self esteem regarding my looks but it was also humiliating because they only saw me from the outside. I was immediately placed into a drug addict, male prostitute category when people would look at me and this was difficult to take. I tried to listen to the advice of Desiree and Cindy and not let it bother me but the truth was, people would feel free to just walk up and grab me even away from work in the most inappropriate places.

One afternoon, I was at a luncheon to celebrate my new boss's promotion to Vice President of Human Resources. I walked into the bathroom and as I walked through the door and turned to use the urinal, I saw a man washing his hands. He looked in the mirror, nodded and smiled. I immediately thought he looked familiar but I didn't know where I could have seen him before. He was a heavy-set man with dark hair and the thing that stood out to me the most was the huge fat roll that was above his shirt collar.

I unzipped my pants and started to relieve myself when I heard him moving. I assumed he was exiting the bathroom since he had just dried his hands.

Thinking nothing of it I continued when all of the sudden, I saw one arm come rushing by my head and another one grabbing my penis. He caused me to pee all over my dress pants because when he grabbed me, it was as if he was trying to rip it off of my body.

I immediately froze and thought, *what in the hell have you gotten yourself into!*

Caught off guard, I couldn't really decide what to do.

I heard him say in a deep raspy voice with a Latin type accent, "You are the little slut tease that is always dancing on those speakers aren't you. I would recognize that ass anywhere."

I couldn't respond initially. I was frozen and panicked. I had never imagined I would find myself in this type of situation by agreeing to work for Cindy.

Finally I said, "I'm not sure what speakers you're talking about, I work in Human Resources at Disney. We are here celebrating my boss's promotion."

Hoping that would be enough to have him question his decision I remained still, trying not to breathe and praying someone would walk in at any minute.

I couldn't even remember his face when I had walked in. I could tell as he continued to press his body up against mine, he was grossly overweight. I felt his sweat smear up against me as he rubbed his face along the back of my neck while he inhaled, smelling my skin.

I wanted someone to open the bathroom door and to get him off of me but at the same time I didn't because I didn't want anyone to believe I was having gratuitous sex in the bathroom with this grotesque man.

He had me pinned between the urinal and his body weight; there was a divider to my left and a wall to my right. He moved his left arm off of the wall and started to place it around my neck like a choke hold.

Finally, I had enough and with all of my strength I pushed off of the edges of the urinal. He lost his footing and staggered back a few steps enough for me to zip my pants up. I turned around and looked at him with the meanest face I could form. I didn't want him for one minute to believe he had scared me.

It was as if the reality of what he had done was even unbelievable to him. He almost seemed embarrassed, as if it was a day dream he was thinking about instead of something he had actually done. He looked at me and quickly scurried out of the bathroom without saying a word.

I walked over to the sink and looked at my khaki pants that were now wet with urine.

How am I going to go out there and explain this? What if I go out there and he is sitting near us in the restaurant? Should I tell management what just happened or will it have the people I work with view me in a different light?

I decided that the best way to hide the urine was to wet a paper towel and blend in all of the water streaks. *I will just tell everyone that the sink faucet squirted all over me when I turned it on.* I looked at the nozzle to see if I could partially unscrew it just in case they questioned me. As soon as I went to try and make the first twist to loosen it someone walked in. Not knowing him, I just looked at him and said, "Don't use that sink, the nozzle on it is broken." He furrowed his brow as he looked at my pants and proceeded to the toilet with a door.

I guess he thought I was some crazy person because I was perched up against the counter, my pants were soaking and I was trying to take the faucet completely off of the sink when he entered. Laughing at myself, something horrible had quickly changed to something comical. I looked down at my pants and it would appear to others as if I had pulled my pants out of the washing machine without drying them.

Arriving back at my table, one of my coworkers looked at my pants and exclaimed, "What happened to your pants," as she pointed, laughed and did everything possible to bring attention to me.

I sheepishly said, "Oh, the faucet in there kind of exploded on me," and I quickly slid back into my chair.

Starring only at my plate, I was fearful to make eye contact with anyone at the table and even more than that, I was afraid that if this guy were to see me again, it would be horrifying if he were to say something to me in front of all of the people I worked with. I kept thinking to myself, *just get through the lunch and then figure out what you need to do later.*

I didn't want to get hung up on what had just happened because developing my career was too important. I needed to keep the secret of my part time job hidden.

That evening I realized the impact of what had actually happened earlier. This man could have killed me and no one would have been the wiser.

I had started doing a bit of traveling and dancing in other bars in Jacksonville, Pensacola and Tampa, but I just didn't want to get pulled into this type of a lifestyle because it was too dangerous. I knew that in time my looks would fade but that an education was something that could never be taken away and if I had to go into debt it was safer than what I was experiencing.

I was creating a chaotic world around me and it went against everything I had worked so hard to get away from. I was trying my attempt at independence and defaulting into an old comfort zone. I was treating myself with the same exploitation that was forced upon me as a child and I realized I was not respecting myself by continuing down this path. I had started skipping classes and calling in sick to work from being so tired from the weekend. I thought that money was the answer to all of my academic problems.

That same Friday night, I went into the club and headed directly to Cindy's office. She was sitting behind her desk, going through some photos.

I knocked on the door frame and she looked up and said, "Hey, I am so glad you are here. You must have been reading my mind. There is a big party that is happening tomorrow night and they asked if they could hire three of our better dancers. I offered you up as one, Patrick and Brandon."

Not looking at her while she was telling me this, I started my rehearsed conversation, "Cindy, I want to thank you so much for this opportunity, but I have to be honest. This is not the type of life I really want to have." Realizing that it had sounded much better in my head I began to fumble over my words, "It's not that there is anything wrong with this type of life, I just want more than dancing on a speaker." Feeling as if I was digging myself into a deeper hole rather than making things better, I fumbled on, "I guess what I am trying to say is that school is the most important thing to me right now and..."

She interrupted me and with a smirk on her face softly said, "I knew it was short lived for you. I know what you are trying to say and I appreciate you so much for sticking it out as long as you have."

I couldn't believe how remarkable she was. She was always caring but she also held true to what she did. She respected me but at the same time took her job very serious. "I have already given the coordinator of that party your name; can you do this one last gig for me?"

I was hesitant to say yes because I just wanted things to go back to normal and I wanted to start regaining my self-respect, but because she was so wonderful and accommodating of me I couldn't let her down. "Sure, but this will be my very last time."

"Thank you," she exclaimed as she jumped up from her chair. She walked around to the front of the desk and put her hands on my cheeks. "I am so proud of you, I hope you know how special you are and if anyone ever tells you differently let me know and I will kick their ass," she said as she wrapped her arms around me and kissed me on the cheek.

She pulled herself away and quickly reminded me, "Now you agreed to work the party tomorrow night right?"

Laughing, I replied, "Yes but this is the last time. No more okay?"

She smiled and softly tapped my cheeks as if she were my grandmother and said, "Thank you sweetie, you will have a blast there and make some great money. We are covered here for tonight so why don't you go on home. I'll get all of the details and confirm with them and get the information to you tomorrow."

The next day came and it was wonderful. I had gone to bed early and woken up early for the first time on the weekend since I had started dancing. I had forgotten how much I loved hearing the day wake up, hearing people out on their morning runs, walking their dogs, the birds chirping in the trees.

I was savoring a cup of coffee when I felt the universe shift. It was like a wave of reality rushing through my head. I could see myself living the absolute perfect life. Making money, living in a beautiful home, and experiencing healthy happy relationships with people around me that were loving and supportive. It was as if the vision was so powerful and obvious that everything I had ever worried about before was just a waste of energy. I knew that what I dreamed would be what I got if I held true to what I wanted.

I was beginning to regret agreeing to dance at the party that Cindy had booked because I really didn't want to go. I felt I owed her the favor but I was getting back to a place where I felt I owed me more things than I owed to others. I didn't want to renege on the obligation and I certainly didn't want to burn any bridges. I didn't understand I was being too nice for my own good.

That evening came and just as she had mentioned, Cindy called and gave me all of the details for going to the party. I was to meet the other two dancers, Patrick and Brandon, there. I had no idea what they looked like or who they were. The only person I had really worked with was Desiree and I was not even sure that was her real name.

I followed the directions that led me about an hour outside of Orlando to a town called Apopka. I found the house set back off of the road about a hundred yards. It was so dark it was almost impossible to make out the size, color or layout from the outside. I pulled down the long driveway and parked at the edge of the house. I didn't want to be blocked in and I couldn't find another place to park that allowed for me to leave easily.

I got my things out of the back seat and walked to the door. I could hear the music as I got closer and the voices were very loud. People were laughing and screaming over one another to have a conversation. It was only ten thirty and the party sounded as if it had been going on for hours.

I knocked three times and stood there for about a minute waiting for someone to answer the door. I then rang the doorbell a series of times and knocked on the door again. Suddenly, the door flung open and an older aged drunk man slurred, "You must be the third guy." His accent was a sickening deep southern aristocrat exaggerated sound overemphasizing every syllable. He continued and it would have been preferable to hear fingernails down a chalk board. "The others are in here sweetheart so why don't you just bring your things and join 'em."

He led me to a bedroom that was just to the left of the front door. When I walked in I saw two other guys that I recognized. They were both sitting Indian style on the floor and looked like they were bobbing for apples with a ten dollar bill shoved up their nose followed by a quick and fast, sniffing sound.

I looked at them, and thought *oh, my God, I really don't want to be here. If something else comes up that I don't like or agree with I am out of here.*

I looked at the guys and nodded my head, "what's up." Walked to the corner of the bedroom and got changed. We were asked to bring only shorts and boots to dance in so getting changed only took about a minute. I was standing there doing some sit ups before we were supposed to go outside as the same guy that answered the door came walking in.

"Now, I want you boys to be as nasty as you want to because today is Hussein's birthday."

I had no idea who this guy was. I knew that the two guys bobbing for cocaine were Patrick and Brandon but I didn't know which one was which. The urge to leave was becoming more and more intense. Trying not to let Cindy down, I thought it would be nice to know who Hussein was so we could make sure we gave him extra attention. I asked the guy in a flirtatious way to start kicking off the illusion of thinking he was sexy, "Can you show me which one he is so I can make sure we give him the extra attention he deserves on his birthday."

With an almost demonic look on his face he said, "Now you're talking sweetness, come over here and let me point him out."

I walked over to the door and looked between the crack and he pointed and said, "That is him right there."

I could see a guy sitting down in a club chair. There were so many people around him it was hard to determine exactly what he looked like so I continued to glare until I could get a good visual. As soon as the path cleared, I could make his face out.

Oh my God, I uttered to myself. It was the same guy that had cornered me in the bathroom.

How did I wind up here? Of all the places in Orlando to be what are the odds that I would be the one selected to come to this party?

I looked at the guy at the door, turned and looked that the two other guys and said, "I can't do this," I said with venomous fury coming from my voice.

"That bastard cornered me in the bathroom earlier this week and I am not interested." I was throwing my things into my bag as I talked. I looked over at the guys wiping the powder from their noses and said, "If you talk to Cindy tell her I'm sorry but this is not my thing."

The old man that had just shown me who Hussein was stood in the door way with his arms extended to each side thinking he could block me. He was about five-feet-six inches and I guess he thought his money made him strong.

"You aren't going anywhere," he said in his condescending accent. "He knew that was you in the bathroom and that is why I called Cindy to make sure you would be one of the guys here tonight. I paid for your ass tonight so it's mine. You walk yourself back over there and put your bag down."

I was not sure if he understood how stupid he sounded so I curled my lip as if I had just smelled the most grotesque odor in the world, rolled my eyes and pushed him out of the way. I pushed him with such force that he crashed into the table that was right beside the front door and I went storming out to my car.

He came running behind me screaming, "I paid good money for you so you can't leave." I stopped mid stride and angrily spun around obviously startling him. It was as if a holographic image of Pop had appeared and the rage grew within me. Then without any intention of stopping, I released this anger that flew from me like a dragon blowing fire.

"You need to understand something you drunk bastard, I am not a consumer good, I am a human being. It is illegal in the state of Florida to purchase people so unless you want me to call the cops, I suggest you walk your ass back inside and tell your sadomasochistic birthday boy to go to hell. Oh, and tell him the money he spent tonight is for him grabbing me in the bathroom," I turned back and threw my things into the car, slammed my door and spun out driving down the long driveway back to Orlando.

I started to recap the night on my drive home. My heart began to sink.

Cindy knew about this all along and she also knew the type of situation I was going to be putting myself in. I guess she is a business woman even at the expense of others safety. She had to have known when they asked for three guys they were referring to me. If not how would the guy have known who I was? How would he have known Cindy?

I guess it really doesn't matter anymore and the lesson in this is honoring what I feel. If I had stayed there out of obligation then who knows what would have happened to me. Cindy was only worried about getting paid, not my well being. This proves once again that the only person I can trust is me. I love me more than anybody else, and I need to be sure I never forget that.

CHAPTER 13

GRADUATION DAY

When I began to think about what I was going to do after college, I was petrified. For ten years of my life I had been working as hard as I possibly could to graduate. I was scared because I didn't know what I would do now that I had invested all of that work and effort into my education.

What would I do if I didn't make it? It is unthinkable for me to go this far and not make it.

There was no more driving up and down the East West Expressway paying tolls every day. No more fighting to get the schedule I needed to accommodate my classes, no more late- night cram sessions, or waking up early to study after getting home at three in the morning. It also meant an end to a world that I had grown accustomed to and that I'd have to adjust to completely different types of stress that awaited me in the unknown.

I decided that since I was graduating, it was time to make a bold move. I wanted to go where I thought jobs were plentiful and where people were diverse. It wasn't that I didn't love Orlando but I was convinced I just needed something more if I wanted to make it. I had made several trips to New York City to get familiar with it and had fallen in love with the city. It seemed that everything began and ended there.

The energy of the city was something I had never experienced. I would look around and often think, *what in the world would Nelly say to me about doing this?* She would most likely say, "keep on going and don't stop. Life is just too short to stop accomplishing the things God has given to you."

I had made some wonderful new friends and contrary to popular belief, the people there were refreshingly honest and nice. That helped me make my final decision. I sold everything I had in Orlando to prepare for my move to New York City the day after graduation.

I will never forget the day itself; it was Saturday August 8, 1998, my college graduation day. I was very excited and most of my family was attending. My mother, sister, cousins, aunts, and uncles all came out to celebrate with me. Dad and Samantha were there as well. It was the first time since Evelyn's wedding that we'd all been together in one place, and I was praying it wouldn't turn into another one of the nightmare days my family was famous for.

Frankly, I was selfish enough to want the entire day to be focused on me. This was my day and, regardless of what everyone else may say or do, that was the whole point of the day. I had worked ten long years all by myself, but more than that, in those years I had learned a great deal about myself and my capabilities.

I was the first person in my family to graduate from college, which was both a good thing and a bad thing. It was good because I persevered and obtained the goal I had set for myself, beating the odds against me and even overcoming the lack of support I received from everyone. The bad thing is that since I earned my degree in Psychology, I learned a great deal about them and how unhealthy their behavior was. To have them close to me in my life would mean that I would choose to either remain unhealthy or choose to separate as far as I could while I continued to work on me. I determined that regardless of what took place, I was going to have a magnificent day.

I woke up that Saturday morning and thought how incredible it was that I didn't have to go back to campus again unless I wanted to. I was done with classes and ready to start a new stage of my life. I walked into the kitchen and got a cup of coffee and started looking around the apartment.

Walking through each room, I reminisced about the people I'd met and learned to love and fear in Orlando. I had loved this apartment from the moment I laid eyes on it. A friend had told me about it and gone with me to see it the first time.

It was on the top floor of a house that had been divided into two apartments and a studio. It was in a desirable part of downtown, on the corner of Livingston and Summerlin Avenues. Though I wasn't sure what to expect, the minute we pulled into the driveway, I knew it was the place I wanted to live.

Entering the driveway, you passed under a porte-cochere. The house was white with blue trim and looked huge from the outside. We parked the car and headed to the front porch. Walking up the three steps and through the creaky screen door I saw the beautiful red Spanish tile and the archways that outlined the front of the house and were covered with screen to protect you from insects. Then as I turned I saw three doors. The door on the left was for the downstairs apartment and the door on the right led to the very small studio apartment. The middle door led to the apartment that would be available as soon as the couple moved out.

We rang the doorbell and a voice from upstairs yelled for us to come in. When we opened the door, I looked up at a hardwood banister that circled the edges at the top of the landing. Walking up the stairs, each step had its own unique sound. The landing at the top had a gorgeous sitting area, and I was immediately enraptured. I started to get butterflies in my stomach because it was almost too good to be true that I could live in something so beautiful.

To the right of the landing was a kitchen. It was huge, with a bar, room for a breakfast table and a storage closet. I turned to my left and saw the living room that was equally impressive. There was a bedroom in front of the house and a master bedroom in back, with a bathroom beside the living room. There were hardwood floors in every room but the kitchen. I was more than amazed!

I didn't want to appear too excited because I knew the couple leaving had mixed feelings about moving, but I also knew I couldn't wait to be living here. The house was within walking distance of downtown and one of the city's most beautiful lakes, where there was always something going on.

Within a week, I was living in that beautiful apartment, and I had been there for eight years. I remembered the various roommates who had come and gone and wondered how I made it through all of them. Some I knew and some were friends of friends that needed some help. My best times were when I lived there alone and the apartment came alive to shield me, keep me company and tell me stories that I made up in my head about all of the people that had lived there before me.

I showered and got dressed for the biggest event of my life. We arrived early and I was thrilled Margaret had made it up from Panama City to see me graduate. She was my sanity check while my family was around. Since she was a neutral party and not involved in any familial issues, I rode with her to the stadium so we could laugh together and I could tell her how important she was to me for being so loyal over the years. I was so excited she'd taken the time out of her busy schedule to share this day with me. It was important she were there to signify the beginning of the dream and the ending of the accomplishment.

We pulled into the parking lot and it was already getting full. We had to park out on a grass lot and walk towards the entrance. I left her when we reached the stadium doors and promised to find her after the ceremony.

The stadium was brand new and huge. When it wasn't being used for an event like this, it was the school's basketball stadium. It was incredible how many people it could hold. I followed the alphabet signs posted on the wall of a long corridor that led to a room where volunteers were sitting to give us instructions on what to do next.

They handed us a card to verify our names and what our degree was in and once we signed off, we were led to a line of people that were preparing to be seated. We were told to walk in single file and get into our seats so that the ceremony would run smoothly and people would be walking up one behind the other instead of randomly.

We entered the auditorium on the bottom floor and as we walked out you could see rows and rows of folding chairs facing the stage which was set for us to walk across and receive diplomas. The stadium seats were filled with families and friends there to celebrate with the people graduating and you could hear the murmur of their voices. I felt as if I couldn't breathe because it was almost too impossible to consider.

We filed in, one behind the other, and as we started the crowd gave us all a standing ovation. I could feel goose bumps start to rise all over my body.

Then I thought, *if they don't call my name I will be so upset.*

I had no reason to think that they wouldn't, it was just almost too hard to believe I had made it to this day.

Typical of a graduation ceremony, it was long and tedious and the anticipation of them reaching my name was becoming more intense as they got further along in the alphabet. I listened as they called everyone's name, and my classmates walked up, one by one, to receive their degrees.

Overcome by a flood of emotions, I attempted to suppress my tears of joy. I was older than most of the other graduates sitting around me and I didn't want to make a fool of myself. Regardless of how hard I tried to focus on something else, I couldn't stop recalling what I had done to make it to this point. Flashing in my mind was the conversation I had with Dad and Samantha and them telling me I was too stupid for college.

Then came the thought about Pop doing all that he could do to make my life hell and unsuccessful. Of course, I also remembered the odd jobs and awkward situations I had put myself in to afford to continue my education. Then the grounding reality of the reason why I did this put it all into perspective. I got my degree not only to further myself, but also to learn about who I am. All of these years, I have worked so hard to dedicate myself to getting better mentally. Finally realizing what has happened to me can only define who I am if I allow it to.

I lost my childhood because of Pop and now I sacrificed a great deal of my young adulthood to focus on getting this diploma and healing. While the names were being read in the background, I looked around the room at all of the parents there to support their children. I wondered absently how many of them had no idea how lucky they were to have their parents pay for their education or how great it was to be skilled enough to receive a scholarship because of sports, academia or whatever other means they used. Then as I focused on the faces sitting beside me I began to wonder if they too had hidden stories about how they were able to make it to this gateway of their life.

I was trying to remain stoic but could feel the uncontrollable drops of emotion rolling down my cheeks. I was so proud of myself and all I had achieved. I knew this was only the first step of many of my accomplishments. I was not prepared for tears running down my face. I never expected this would be my reaction.

Until they called my name, I remained in doubt of graduating. I was going back through everything I could recall that might hinder my name not being called: *do I have any overdue library books, fees I may have forgotten, campus parking tickets I had received?*

I wanted to make sure all these things had been handled in the correct manner. I had receipts so I was positive there were no outstanding financial debts I owed to the school, but I was still nervous that my name wouldn't be called.

As they finally got to the letter G, I heard them call my name; the tears were rolling down my face again. I was embarrassed but at the same time I didn't care anymore. I went up to the stage and shook the hands of the dean and president of the school as they congratulated me.

As I left the stage, a photographer snapped a picture, capturing the expression on my face as I fully realized the success of the goal that was thought by so many to be unachievable.

I returned to my seat and let out a huge sigh of relief. Mentally, I placed a huge checkmark beside my biggest triumph that I'd been told I'd never do. I let my thoughts drift and began to wonder what I would do now. My whole life had been focused on college, and it was slightly unsettling to know that big objective was no longer out there in front of me.

What would my next accomplishment be in life? I hadn't thought beyond this day. The only thing I had prepared for me next was moving to New York. Would I have a family, stay single, get a job that would exercise my creativity and challenge me all at the same time? I had no idea, but one thing that I knew for sure was that regardless of what else may happen to me, I had my degree. My childhood had been taken, but this is something no one could ever take away from me.

After the ceremony, I went to thank Dad and Samantha for coming. Most people could do that with the entire family present at an event like this, but I had to sneak around to the back of the building and meet them separately so Mom wouldn't get mad at me for speaking to them first.

As I rounded the back of the building and saw them standing there, I couldn't stop my rush of satisfaction. We hugged and they congratulated me, telling me how proud they were. Samantha exhibited her usual grace by saying she didn't want to interfere with plans I had with Mom, but she wouldn't have missed seeing the ceremony today for anything in the world. I understood completely why she said that, and after a brief conversation, we went our separate ways.

I hurried to the front of the building to pretend I'd been looking for Mom and the rest of my family. It seemed foolish, but I knew it was the best way to handle these circumstances. When I spotted them, they were waiting for me as a group at the front entrance. Everyone expressed their pride in me, and I felt liberated, knowing how hard I had worked to gain control of my life and achieve this feat.

After the adrenaline of graduation started to wear off, uncertainty began to settle over me. Back at my apartment, I looked at everything I had accumulated and realized I was getting ready to put this part of my life behind me. I was nervous and excited at the same time. I knew that if I could make it through the rigorous demands of working and college that I could undoubtedly make it in New York.

It was then when I saw a piece of red fabric sticking up from one of the boxes. Not able to recall packing anything red, I reached in and pulled out the red velvet comforter that Mama'O had made for me. It was as if someone had given me a super hero cape. I remembered all of the nights I had this beautiful velvet cloak shielding off all evil and dangers I could think of. With this shield in my hand and all of the Angels I had over me it reminded me I wasn't alone.

My good friend Marcar was letting me live with him until I got on my feet and found a place to live. He and I had met while I was working at Disney World. He was very extroverted and loved talking to people. The two of us had hit it off really well. He was from Brazil and had a beautiful apartment on the corner of 86th Street and Central Park West. It overlooked Central Park and reminded me of an apartment you'd see in a television show based in New York. Things were falling into place perfectly. I packed the rest of my life into six boxes, hoping I had everything I needed to live in a place like New York City.

I took my boxes to the shipping store and completed the forms to mail them. I grunted as I picked the boxes from the floor onto the scale.

The UPS clerk acknowledged, "These boxes sure are heavy,"

"I know. My entire life is in these is boxes," I said and sent them on their way. A few days later, Marcar called to let me know everything arrived in good condition. I told my family I was headed to the Big Apple and had great expectations about living there. I was sure I would find an incredible job, live in a huge apartment, and make more money than I'd ever made in my life. I knew I was in for a real treat.

My friends threw a going-away party for me the evening before I left. It was an electrifying and emotional evening because I truly cherished the friends I'd made in Orlando. They had helped me grow and mature, giving me the support I needed to be a healthy, competent adult. I looked around at the people that I had befriended and realized how diverse they all were. Bankers, Real Estate Brokers, waiters, drag queens, straight, gay, rich, poor and of every culture and race were giving me the send off party of a life time.

I couldn't believe the turnout and how many people that had touched my life. Some of them were excited for me; others were scared for me, but they all supported my decision to uproot and move on. I woke up the next morning feeling I was facing a new day that would change my life forever. I gathered the few things I had left to take with me and packed my suitcase. With butterflies in my stomach, I did one last walk around the apartment.

While I was wondering what it would be like living in New York City, I had a moment of panic, thinking I was making a huge mistake. It was too late to change my mind; however, I had to follow through on my commitment.

With a final deep exhale, I grabbed my suitcase and headed down the stairs for the last time. At the front door, I glanced back at the home that had brought me so much peace and safety and had become the place where I truly grew up. I then closed the door ending that chapter of my life. Walking under the archway to the back parking area, I loaded my suitcase into the trunk of the car and headed off to the airport. Pulling out of the driveway, I continued to think how wonderful my life had been there and how grateful I was for all the experiences I had enjoyed.

CHAPTER 14

SURRENDERING IN NEW YORK

The flight to New York was uneventful but I was still mourning leaving my life in Orlando behind trying to decide why I wanted to start a new life somewhere else. I had elected to leave everything that was familiar to me but I didn't know why.

Was it because I needed to experience new things? Then it hit me, *it was because I don't want to become content and stagnant with the time I had. I want to continue to push myself to achieve new things. I don't want to be complacent and maintain the same life. I want to experience everything fully. While I appreciate and love everyone that was in my life, I needed to push ahead.*

I was mentally exhausted by the time we landed at LaGuardia Airport. I got off of the airplane and looked through the crowd and, true to his nature; Marcar was standing there with a welcoming smile. He began telling me all the things we would be doing, and it immediately put me at ease. We went to the baggage claim, where I retrieved my suitcase, and we headed through the door to a taxi. Sitting in the cab, heading to Marcar's apartment, I found myself wondering, *what have I done? I feel more intimidated than I have in years. I thought I would be better once we started driving and the sight of the city became home but I didn't.* It took me a few minutes to remind myself, *I am a fighter and I can handle anything out there. I am strong, independent and ready for a new life. My fears will not be my reality.*

It seemed as if I was in a different country not a different city and state. My first surprise came when I discovered Marcar's building had a doorman. I didn't realize the significance of that in the beginning. Apparently a building with a doorman sends the message that this is a nice place, and the prices are a little higher. I had brought two thousand dollars with me, thinking that would be enough to get me into an apartment.

The fact was the apartment I had been paying four hundred dollars for in Orlando had been a dream deal. I had asked Marcar on several occasions about rent, and he had assured me it was comparable to Orlando. What I didn't realize was his idea of money was somewhat skewed because he lived off a trust fund and thought nothing of paying fifteen hundred dollars a month for an apartment.

I was elated to discover that the people Marcar hung out with seemed to care for one another like a family. I was looking forward to making new friends and getting to know as much about New York City as I could. I immediately began looking for work, and I realized that the competition was fiercer than I thought it would be.

Apparently everyone in New York was looking for a job. I was not sure what I had gotten myself into and it wasn't long before I discovered I was truly frightened about my living situation. I couldn't live with him forever but I was almost out of my money.

Marcar and I attended a party where I met some incredible people. I remember looking around the room and thinking this was why I had moved. I was standing in a circle of people from Brazil, Russia, Paris, and Nebraska, and then there was little ole me from Florida. I was actually kind of surprised I could handle conversations with so many people from different places around the world.

As I made my way through the crowd, I met several people who spoke multiple languages. I was intrigued and petrified at the same time and knew I was definitely out of my league. I spoke English and Spanish, but not on the same level. These people glided seamlessly from French to English to Spanish without pausing to think. I quickly felt they were much higher caliber people than I was.

I fought the vulnerable feelings that started to re-surface like it had done so many years ago. I had worked hard to overcome these insecurities but the reality was, I didn't do away with them, I had just dealt with them in the particular moment. Different environments and situations were causing me to go into a spin.

It took a few weeks, but I finally got a job with a recruiting firm. When they asked if I was interested in a job, I was ecstatic because the only other offer I'd had was to be manager of a pizza restaurant where I'd get paid under the table if I kept quiet about the adult film business in the back room.

I was excited to have a new job and I thought I'd be getting on my feet and starting my real life in New York City soon. However, I continued to be intimidated by the people around me, and I was becoming consumed with this insecurity. I realized all the issues I had spent years working through during college were returning with a vengeance. I'd find myself at parties, gravitating to the corner where I felt ready to cry, wanting to become invisible. Prior to this, I was the life of the party and people sought me out for entertaining conversations. I was becoming withdrawn and antisocial. There were even times when I thought it would be easier to kill myself.

The feelings of abuse were resurfacing, and I once again doubted my capabilities. I spent many sleepless nights worrying that I would never be good enough to do what I needed to do. It literally took me hours to decide what to wear that looked good and made me feel good about myself. I usually ended up borrowing clothes from Marcar because I thought my clothes weren't good enough.

I thought I had overcome what the abuse had done to me, but that was far from the truth. I had misled myself down an invented path believing I was "cured" and I had gotten over the abuse and it's effects on me. I felt like I was right back where I was the day I'd turned Pop in to the police.

I was struggling to decide where I fit in the world, and I had once again put myself into a situation I didn't know how to get out of.

I ended up resigning from the job I thought would change my life. I had been assigned to a sales role on the Portuguese side of the business and couldn't speak the language. Though I could speak Spanish, it didn't translate well into Portuguese. I made unintentional sexual propositions, while telling people I was a crazy goat. A favorite example of mine that reflected my inability to speak Portuguese was the initial greetings I used with customers. When the greeting was translated it meant, *I thought their fat blow job was a mother.* It was mutually agreed upon that I wasn't a good fit for the job.

For the second time in my life, I had no control over my destiny. I had no money for rent or food and no job prospects on the horizon. Fortunately, I was with wonderful people who continued to provide a place for me to live and food so I didn't go hungry. More than anything, I didn't want to be a failure. I didn't know what to do next and felt completely at a loss. I had been in New York City for almost a year, and the six boxes that had been my life were now reduced to a green army duffle bag that I carried from place to place with all my worldly possessions as I stayed with one friend and another. This was not what I had envisioned for my life at all, and I knew it was time to make some changes.

I finally gave in to the chaos in my mind, and the insecurities I was filled with became too much for me to deal with. They were impeding my ability to make simple decisions about my survival.

Dad and Samantha were coming to Buffalo, New York, to visit her sister for Christmas.

I desperately needed to hear a familiar voice, so I called them collect from a phone booth on the street corner. I was afraid that Dad would view me as a failure and never do anything to help me out but I had to give it a try. I picked up the receiver and I could feel the winter freeze from the hard plastic penetrate through my glove. I pressed zero and waited for the operator to answer. Almost immediately I heard a voice say, "Operator."

I knew it was something I had to do. I couldn't turn back now. "Yes, I would like to make a collect call."

I trusted I had the right number for Samantha's sister. She had given it to me before I moved just in case I needed to get in touch with someone close by. The operator responded back in her rote tone, "Name please," That was the most horrific question. I didn't want her to announce my name to Samantha's family as a collect caller but at the same time I knew it was just a matter of days before I was truly homeless again. I hoped that this didn't embarrass them too much but I couldn't think of an alternative.

"Yes, ma'am, my name is Grant." I wanted to go on and explain to her to ask for Dad when she called but her tone was so dismissive that I would be lucky if she got my name right for them to accept the charges.

I heard Samantha's sister answer and then the operator say, "I have a collect call from Grant, do you accept the charges?" That question alone was one of the most shameful questions I had heard since my arrival. I wanted to hear her say "yes" so badly but I also wanted to hang up because I was so embarrassed I didn't have enough money to pay for the call.

As always, she was wonderfully polite and accommodating. She responded to the operator, "Oh, of course we do."

The call was connected and I was not prepared to speak with her. I had been rehearsing in my mind what I would be saying to Dad. I heard the operator drop off of the line, then immediately followed the alerted sounding question, "Hey Grant are you doing okay? Do you want me to get your Dad for you?" It was as if she already knew I was waving my white flag of defeat.

I didn't want to alarm her but I was desperate to talk to Dad, "I'm fine, but yes I would really like to speak with him if he is around."

Without hesitation and sounding as if she were already in motion as her volume decreased while saying, "Hold on let me get him for you."

I could hear her yelling his name in the background. Then the movement of her phone created a muffled noise and then bursting onto the line was Dad, "Hello?" I didn't know what to say. My tone was meek and my voice was filled with defeat as I said, "Dad, I'm not going to make it here. I really need some help."

When I decided to call him, I had no idea the conversation would feel so reminiscent of the day I hide behind the General Store meat counter in Gulf Shores fourteen years ago. That day, I knew Dad would know what to do, and I felt the same way standing on the street corner in New York City. The cold air whizzing around me and all the fight I had left in me was completely gone.

With a very understanding tone and most of all, comforting, he said, "I understand. Why don't you come up to Buffalo and meet us for Christmas and then move to Atlanta with us? I know you'll love it there. It is a big city and filled with people your age. It is one of the largest cities in the South and a place I know you will fit in."

It sounded as if he too had been rehearsing this conversation for a while.

I was so relieved and overjoyed, tears filled my eyes and it was as if a huge weight was lifted from my shoulders. I was barely able to talk as my tears turned to uncontrollable weeping. Without even trying to sound prideful I simply said, "Okay."

That's it, okay? No questions, I thought.

I continued, trying to talk through the hyperventilating and my now frozen lips. "Dad, thank you for always being there for me, I'm so scared and didn't know what to do. Thank you so much"

We worked out the details and tenderly hung up the phone and placed my head on the back of my hand that was still clutched to the phone as it rest in the cradle. I composed myself as best I could by taking a few deep breaths. I reached down and put my duffle bag that contained my possessions that were now almost nothing over my shoulder, turned and walked down the sidewalk. All I wanted to do was get to a place where I felt protected.

Dad told me he would wire me money for a train ticket to Buffalo, and he then buy me a plane ticket to Atlanta.

I went running to the store to get the money that he had wired and headed off to Penn Station to buy my train ticket. The train was leaving at one twenty and I was standing in the purchase line. I had never been there before and I had no idea what I was supposed to do. It was already twelve forty and I didn't want to get on the wrong train and end up somewhere else in the North East.

What happened next was something surreal. It was as if Nelly could feel what I was going through all over again because out of the blue a lady walked up to me and said, "Looks like you need some help with something." I thought she was someone that worked for the Transit Authority but was just out of uniform. She was short, older but you could tell in her younger years she must have looked like Marian Anderson, the Opera Singer from the thirties. Her accent told me that she had lived in the New York area most, if not all, of her life.

I looked at her and it was like I was seeing Nelly. My mouth was ajar as I looked at her in disbelief. "Yes, I am trying to get on a train to go see my family in Buffalo and I really don't know what to do."

She grabbed my hand and started pushing through the line screaming at everyone, "Move out of my way, this man has to get home to see his family, now come on people let me through."

It was like she was running for a touchdown and refused to let anyone stop her. She pulled me up to the front of the ticket line. I handed her my money to give to the ticket agent, she snatched the ticket out of the agents hand and I thought she would hand it over to me and then direct me to where I needed to go.

She was on a mission and it was making sure I got on that train. She turned and looked back at me and said, "Now, hurry up, pick up your bags and follow me. These platforms can be confusing."

I didn't know what to make of it so I followed her instructions. She had nothing to gain by me getting boarded on time.

We heard the announcement for the final boarding call for the train I was to be leaving on. She started screaming as we approached the platform, "You better hold that train; this boy needs to get to see his family for the holiday." I didn't have the time to tell her that it wasn't just for the holidays but for some reason I think she already knew.

We made it to the right train and once again I thought that would be the end of it. I looked at her as I went to step up onto the train and stuck my hand out to thank her again for her generosity.

She slapped my hand and said, "Do you think they are going to hold this thing all day? Get your butt in there so we can find your seat." I smiled and thought of Nelly. That is exactly something that she would say to me. We rushed down the aisle with her leading me. She found my seat and said, "You have a great, great time with your family and may God bless you."

I gave her a huge hug and tried to hand her some money which she rejected. "I don't need your money, I need you to sit down and get ready to leave."

I smiled, "God has already blessed me," I said as I turned to put my duffle bag over my seat in the luggage compartment. "If it had not been for you I don't think I would have ever made this train."

I turned back to thank her again for the one hundredth time and she was gone. It was as if she had completely disappeared into thin air. I went to go to the door but the train steward had already closed it. I looked out the window and I could not see her anywhere.

I sat down, closed my eyes and said, "Thank you, God, for my Angel."

I just knew she was sent to me to protect and guide me and that I was being told by the Universe, "Okay, now that you have this New York thing out of your system, let's move on with your life."

During the train ride, I did a lot of soul searching, wondering where I had gone wrong and what I could have done differently. I realized it all went back to understanding yourself and knowing exactly who you are. I felt just as violated after living in New York as I had from Pop. I didn't know how I was going to recover from this bleak experience. I thought I was going to go to the big city and conquer the world. Instead, I learned I had significant limitations and needed to slow down and do things in the proper way.

I wasn't a super hero. I had deluded myself by thinking everything was behind me, and I was strong and mentally healthy. I began to understand that a person never truly recovers from abuse. You have to deal with it every time there are changes in your life. You have to come to terms with yourself in every situation and move through the process of recovery at every level of your life. I was not having a pity party but instead I was realizing that there was still a power over me that I needed to better understand.

I was strong living in Orlando but with different situations come different circumstances and I had not been prepared to cope properly. It was like sending someone to war that had never been through boot camp.

When I arrived in Buffalo, I spent most of my time sleeping. I was exhausted, mentally and physically. Living in New York stripped away every last scrap of my self-esteem along with the self security I had worked on for so many years to build.

Once again, I reveled in the unconditional love displayed in Samantha's family as we enjoyed Christmas in Buffalo.

They were excited to be together and still as supportive and loving of one another as they had always been. Her sister was a very successful and accomplished person. Her husband had worked for the President of the United States; she had been an Attorney at the Department of Interior and now they had a stunning home and two wonderful children. He no longer worked for the President because the term had ended. He found a job at a company which brought them to Buffalo.

One afternoon she found me sitting on the couch in her living room just staring into space. She sat down beside me and gently placed her hand on my thigh. When she spoke, I was shocked out of my reverie.

"I hope you know how much I admire you," she said quietly.

I know I must have looked confused because she smiled and said, "Anyone that sticks with college as long as you did and stayed with it all those years to graduate is someone I admire. I was fortunate enough to have my college paid for, and I can honestly say I wouldn't have finished otherwise. I want you to know I sincerely admire you."

I could hear her words, but I couldn't believe them for some reason. I thought she pitied me. I knew, however, this was very much what Samantha's family did when anyone was experiencing problems. They rallied around once they knew someone needed to be lifted up to their potential.

Because I knew that, her words finally penetrated my dreary thoughts. The last few days in Buffalo I was wishing I could blend into the walls. I was embarrassed, humiliated, and felt like a failure. Hearing this wonderful woman's words changed all that and gave me hope that I could get my life back on track.

Later that week, Dad, Samantha and I boarded the flight from Buffalo to Atlanta. Once we landed, I picked up the duffle bag from the luggage carousel and headed to their car. I didn't know where I'd go from here, but I can say now with absolute certainty that my decision to leave New York City and live with them again was the best decisions of my life.

It changed things in more ways than I could have ever imagined. The scars of the abuse that I went through go so deeply that when I was in New York I had only started the healing process. Once I arrived in Atlanta, I continued the healing process, I became aware that I had not been challenged with adversity enough to know how to keep the walls up when necessary and how to let them down when I needed to.

They generously allowed me to live with them while I pieced things back together for myself. I had made a promise to Samantha that I would be out as soon as I could support myself. I assured her I was ready to get back on my feet, and New York was only a brief setback for me. I started putting out resumes immediately and was soon picked up by a company as a contractor and eventually offered a full-time position working on site for The Coca Cola Company. Though I didn't have an Ivy League education, I continued with my quest to do everything in my power to get a Fortune resume.

CHAPTER 15

Your choice, Victim or Survivor

Twenty two years after I exposed Pop's dirty secret, the therapist I'm seeing currently suggested I create a timeline for my life so I could see, in a linear way, how things had progressed to make me the person I am today.

I felt like the day I'd turned Pop in as a sexual predator was a defining moment for me. That was the day I put as the beginning on my timeline because I felt it was the day I began to clearly define who I was. Thus this book began with that event.

As I worked on the timeline, I remembered the conversation with Mom about Pop getting therapy instead of serving time. I realized no one had ever told me anything else about it, and I wondered if there had been a trial for him. Though it took me two weeks to gather my thoughts and muster my courage, I finally dialed the number for the Selma Police Department to get the facts about my case. The horror came when I realized there were no facts because there had never been a case.

As I contemplate the effects of the momentous decision to turn him in, I realize the impact the abuse had on my life is both a blessing and a curse.

I love who I am today, and would not change one second of my life. I wouldn't want to go through the horrific abuse I experienced again, but I don't want to be a different person than I am today. I am not who I am because of the abuse. I am who I am because of my positive actions and the strength I find in situations and people.

As a teen, I am not sure the counselors really understood me, because they focused on the abuse and placed me in the role of victim. I always made it very clear to them I knew I had been victimized, but I didn't have to feel like a victim in terms of my identity, because I didn't do anything to myself. I refused to feel guilty and ashamed because that monster repeatedly beat and raped me.

As I've written this book, I've realized that sexual abuse is at epidemic levels in our society. From what I've read, as many as sixty percent of convicted sexual offenders are on parole or on probation. I also learned that most of the sexual offenders in prison were abused as children. These horrendous facts helped me understand that I need to tell my story.

Getting my story out was the initial reason for going to the lengths I did to get Pop arrested, to separate myself from my family, and push so hard to be the person I was meant to be before my life was interrupted by his abuse. I was determined there would be no cycle of abuse in *my* family.

When I read more statistics about sexual abuse and children, I was stunned. Estimates are that one in four girls and one in six boys are sexually abused before they reach age eighteen. Almost fifty percent of these victims were abused by a family member. Most of the other victims were abused by someone outside the family who was considered a trusted friend. That means only about ten percent of sexually abused children were attacked by strangers.

The reported numbers for boys is questionable, because culturally it is assumed that boys cannot be victims. There is much more shame that goes into a male admitting they were abused because society teaches that boys should be able to fight for themselves. Also, if they were sexually aroused [an involuntary physical response], then they "must have liked it," which of course is not the case.

What is frightening is that experts believe as many as thirty percent of sexual abuse victims never report the abuse. They simply live with their shameful secret gnawing at them their entire lives. The tragedy is that the shame is not theirs at all, but that their silence ensures the monsters that attacked them never have to pay and allows it to continue.

It is likely that the incidence of sexual abuse could be dramatically reduced if more people and educators were less afraid to have a simple, truthful discussion with children. I have had this difficult talk with both of my sons, not only to be sure they understand who should and should not touch them, but also to be sure any accusations they made would be taken seriously by the adults in their lives.

Like many emotional issues, sexual abuse is not something you can heal and "get over." Often a victim of sexual abuse may actually block entire incidents out of their conscious mind, but it remains a living nightmare, with outward repercussions, in the subconscious. This is exactly what I have experienced and what led me to write this book.

From a child's perspective, telling an adult about sexual abuse is very significant because of the lack of credibility adults often give children. Many times parents <u>choose</u> not to believe their children, for a variety of reasons. They may not want to believe what they are hearing, because it is too horrific to contemplate. Instead, they deny the event took place, which places the burden of proof on the child.

If the abuser is someone close to the parents, they may find it easier to say the child is lying instead of believing that a trusted friend or family member could hurt *their family* this way. Many families, like my own, simply accept it as part of the family structure. The inherently conflict-avoidant nature of human beings is a sad reality in families like mine, and there are many of them. It is simply deemed easier to look the other way than to face the reality, even if it means sacrificing the child. Unreal but all-too-common.

In my case, I was petrified that the people that abused me would follow through on their threats of killing me, my Mom, or throwing me in jail. Is it possible for that person to kill all your teachers and friends? It seems possible when you're in a situation completely out of your control.

For a child, who is unable to rationalize the level of risk they take by coming forth as a victim, it is an enormous challenge. What happens if none of the threats take place but your parents or adults believe you and encourage you to tell the police and authorities? Will you have to testify?

Under normal circumstances, it's often difficult for children to talk to parents about something this intimate. Imagine the fear and discomfort of describing sexual abuse to a room full of strangers. How do you get over *that?*

As a survivor of sexual abuse, I understand the impact all these scenarios can have on a child. When a child is sexually abused, not only is it utterly confusing, it makes you wonder if you can trust any adults. Trust is thrown out of the window along with everything else they ever believed was true.

Though I'm an adult now, every day of my life is still impacted at some level from the abuse I suffered from all of the perpetrators that abused me.

Family members have said, "Why can't you just get over it?"

I wonder if they would tell someone severely disfigured externally from torture and abuse to just get over it and move on. The difference is, with a severely disfigured person; the scars from the torture and pain are clearly evident. Survivors of sexual abuse do not always have visible physical scars, but they're often disfigured emotionally. Abuse is like a forever river constantly running through your soul.

The reality is that I am now a forty-year-old grown man with two beautiful children, and sometimes I am still afraid to go to sleep at night. When I am insecure and feeling vulnerable I will sleep on our couch, even though we have an amazing bed, because I feel that if someone were going to attack me there would only be one way for them to approach. The only way for me to get a good night's sleep is to sit up with my cat Charlie, and nod off completely from exhaustion.

Because of this abuse, I have developed some signs and symptoms of Obsessive Compulsive Disorder, in order to control my life in specific areas. This is common among abuse survivors. Before I leave for the day, our bed has to be made. The pillows on the bed have to be in the same order, and I could spend hours adjusting and re-adjusting them to make sure they are perfect. I will wash dishes in the sink instead of in a dishwasher because I just don't feel that the dishwasher gets them clean. I will, and have, washed dishes until my hands have bled from the constant soaking in the water.

I am hypervigilant if my sons display a lack of integrity and work with balancing this every day. My relationships at work are sometimes challenged by my intuition, which is heightened and fine tuned because of always having to be on alert as a child. Corporate America is filled with political injustice and manipulation, and for me, it is a struggle when it is so apparent that someone is trying to lie and manipulate to get ahead.

The first step a survivor of sexual abuse must take is to learn how to release the shame and to love himself or herself. Once you've restored that love, your self-confidence returns, and you can regain control of your life. I will never forget what happened to me, because it was the most horrific experience I have ever endured, but I did eventually move forward and assume power over my life.

A child should feel protected and safe around adults. Period. Additionally, parents should **know** the people with whom their children interact. Even if someone seems to have the child's best interest at heart, you must analyze and determine if that is part of his or her game to get closer to your child. Most importantly, parents should never, ever hesitate to remove their child from the presence of someone who makes them nervous, or about whom their child displays nervousness or troubling words. No matter the social consequences, instincts rarely fail in these situations. We fail *them*, by not heeding our internal safeguards.

My mother left me alone with a family member who had sexually abused her. She assumed it wouldn't happen to me because I was male. She was horribly mistaken. Perhaps. Or perhaps she was quite aware of the danger and chose to override a mother's natural protective instinct.

Parents, I cannot tell you enough how important it is to be familiar with those who are alone with your children. I have a friend whose son's male sixth-grade teacher began taking a group of boys out for snacks after school. When her son begged to go, she wouldn't let him. The only reason she had for not doing that was an uncomfortable feeling about the teacher. During the summer school break, this particular teacher called to talk with her son, and, again, she refused. Later she learned this teacher was prosecuted for molesting young boys. Follow your instincts. Hurt feelings heal easier than sexual abuse scars.

Know the people with your children. Make unplanned visits to their schools. Don't move into a neighborhood and allow your children to go over to a neighbor's house until you know the parents well. Invite the children to your home instead. Make it a point to teach your children about boundaries and remind them they need to scream as the top of their lungs if *anyone* crosses those boundaries.

Once you are a victim of sexual abuse, you begin a tug of war with what is right and what is wrong. Some victims become extremely introverted and most if not all, have low self-esteem. Many turn to drugs because they do not know how to deal with the abuse and lose themselves in the false euphoria drugs bring. Many hide behind a double life, one that includes normalcy and another one that includes risk.

Even though the abuser was an adult who did this to a child, the victims still feel it was something they could have controlled, and guilt is in the forefront of every situation.

Once victimized, there is a driving want to please everyone because you are afraid of not being liked for who you are. Survivors learn to deal with what has happened and stop blaming themselves, realizing that what happened was out of their control.

If you and your child mutually decide to press charges and prosecute, as I did, understand that it's painful because it is an exercise for healing and learning about respect, not necessarily just for the outcome of the event.

In my case, even though I had six witnesses that wrote letters, the case was thrown out due to lack of evidence. In the small town of Selma, Alabama, where Pop lived, he had deep-rooted political ties, and he was well connected. In my opinion the people that were serving in political office shared the same opinion of supporting segregation and white supremacy by participating in the same civic organizations as him. Because of their brotherhood my case just disappeared.

The irony is that even though the courts did not prosecute him, life did. He spent his entire life building up a family that would idolize and worship him and the reality is that no one in my family gives him any respect. Mema chose not to see what was happening before her and she developed a disease called Retinitis Pigmentosa and gradually lost her sight. Just because you do not get convicted in our legally defined Justice System does not guarantee an existence free of consequences.

If your child comes to you with information like this, you may find it difficult to believe. However, it is important that your support for your child is evident until you are able to discern the truth. Never make your children feel it is wrong to tell you something of this nature. You will earn credibility and respect that will ensure they'll be able to share all their fears with you because you can be trusted.

People do not "get over" being sexually abused, but they can learn to find strength in the adversity of it and realize how liberating and powerful it feels to have the courage to stand up for themselves.

Children learn their behaviors from adult's: parents, teachers, ministers, police officers in their lives. Perpetrators choose these professions so they can prey on children while hiding under the umbrella of their job.

As a parent, you are responsible for your actions and words. Listen to your children, and be your child's advocate. Regardless of whether you're a father, mother, aunt, uncle, preacher, teacher, police officer, brother, neighbor, friend, or babysitter, sexual abuse is *wrong*.

Please empower children to tell adults not to touch them, to help children know how to explain to adults when they feel uncomfortable. Empower your children to feel free to tell anyone in authority what is happening to them. Children are to be protected, molded, nurtured, supported, and above all, not manipulated as adult toys.

Nelly taught me so much, about life and about being seen as less than you are through the self-serving eyes of bigots and racists. I am a better person for knowing and seeing the events that took place in Selma and the South through her eyes.

Both of my sons are adopted and have their own pasts to work on, and because of my experiences, I feel I am better able to help. I look at them and know that there is no way I would knowingly put them at risk. They will never spend the night with or even socialize with someone who has a history or suspicion of neglecting or hurting children.

I also approach their healing from a different perspective than a non-abused parent might. The first time my youngest son looked at me and used the excuse, "You know, I was abused," I looked back at him and said, "I was abused too."

He didn't know what to do; I went on, "Devin, life is full of great things if you choose to accept them. You can choose to sit around a table and tell everyone you were abused. They'll probably feel sorry for you. Personally, I don't want their pity. I have the power to say I was abused, but I am not a victim. I chose not to allow people to keep seeing me as a victim."

Today, Devin will tell you exactly what he feels and then advise you to pick yourself up when you are down. Both of my boys are simply amazing.

After telling mom about what I suffered at the hands of her father, I demanded to go into therapy. The first female therapist I saw asked me a question that changed me forever, "Have you ever had the urge to do this to children yourself?"

I realized then that no one would truly understand my motives or me as long as they saw me through the abuse I suffered. I never had a desire to do to other children what was done to me.

When I asked why she'd asked me that question, she said, "Statistically, you are more likely to become a drug addict, an alcoholic, an underachiever, or even commit suicide because you were sexually abused."

Remembering what Dr. Henderson had told me about the same statistics, I looked at her, and with a voice filled with determination and anger, I said, "Life has given me the opportunity to prove the statistics wrong. After all, I'm as good as the person putting the numbers on the paper. I am not a statistic, I didn't ask to have this happen to me, and I certainly don't believe I am going to become anything other than who I am."

I look at the things that happened to me and thank God I am alive. More than that, I am thankful I am sane and work every day to ensure I keep life in perspective. I think Nietzsche's saying, "What does not kill me makes me stronger," is an accurate statement of my life.

What I know is I am great at being the best I can be for me. I have spent years getting to know myself, understanding and identifying my boundaries. I had to learn what unconditional, healthy love looked like.

Unconditional love is "without condition," and this was one of the hardest things for me to put into practice. I always thought I needed to please others or prove to them that I was worthy. What I didn't realize, until I was in my thirties, is I only needed to prove I was worthy to myself.

I am fortunate. I have an amazing relationship with my partner and my kids. I am the founder of A Village To Raise, www.avillagetoraise.com. It is a social networking website we created for parents with adopted children, children with special needs or families that are defined as non-traditional. I am a successful writer and public speaker and spend as much time as I can, volunteering and being an advocate for adoption, survival of abuse, and parenting.

The definition of a victim can be someone who embraces their misfortune and chooses to stay helpless to change its impact on their life. If you choose to live by this definition, then you choose always to be a victim. My definition of being a victim is not the same. Being a victim to me means I was in a place that created an unfortunate situation for me. I should pull from that what I don't want to be or do and appreciate the lesson and take it forward with me in life.

One of the most difficult days in my life was the call I received from Mom when I was thirty one. I was at work and she called to let me know that Nelly had died. The only person in my life that understood me was suddenly gone. I felt so guilty for not maintaining better communication with her as I was achieving the goals she and I had discussed throughout my life. She continued to talk but I was deaf to her words. I couldn't help but wonder what had really happened to her.

Once the conversation ended I wanted to know for myself that she was really dead. It's not that I didn't believe her, I just needed to know for myself because it would not be the first time someone told me incorrect information about Nelly.

I went to the web page for *The Selma Times Journal* and looked up the obituary section. As I scanned the page I saw her name and my heart sunk. Nelly Johnson. The article said that she died of natural causes but there was no age listed. I am not sure if she even had a birth certificate because I knew she was born in a house, not a hospital. A small summary of who she was survived by was mentioned. What a terrible account of a woman that helped me survive such a horrific childhood. I wanted so badly for my name to be mentioned there as well.

I wish I could share with her today all of the accomplishments I have achieved in my life because I know how proud she would be. She would love my kids as I do, and she would be so excited to know I graduated from college and that I am successful in family, finances, health and spirituality, which was her definition of wealth. She would laugh because the red velvet covers that kept me safe all of these years now cover the chaise lounge chair in my living room. The Chair is now a thing of beauty and is a reminder of the closeness and security she provided me.

Some who read my story may be left with questions about the family members and friends I have described. What became of them? How did it all work out?

I have made the choice not to go into great identifying detail, for several reasons. First and foremost, these are people who have shown drive, determination, and commitment to one dubious cause for the entire length of my life (and theirs): the cover-up of this family secret. Certain members of the family have dedicated themselves to this mission even when it meant the sacrifice of their own children. Their denial is what defines them, and ultimately ruins them.

Naturally, this "denial" is not genuine in the sense of not being able to remember, or of truly believing that my grandfather is innocent. No, just the opposite – they are completely aware and without excuse. The decision to keep silent, and to attack anyone who refuses to be silent, is a conscious choice, an act of will. I am reminded of my Aunt Patricia's words that first day I reported the abuse: "*You are doing the right thing and they are embarrassed that they didn't*". Upon reading this book, their vengeance and their desire to maintain the shreds of their precious public image will, I'm certain, be total.

Therefore, I take little interest in engaging in debate. I have no need to defend the veracity of my words, because no matter their response, the one thing they will never be able to do is to remove the reality from my memory, or from their own. It doesn't work that way.

I will say that my grandfather is still alive, as are most other members of my family, including my grandmother and my parents. I enjoy a close relationship with my stepmother Samantha to this day, and we look forward to the times that she and my father visit us. I do have a relationship with my mother, though her willingness to acknowledge the truth, and her share of the responsibility, fluctuates daily. We do not visit her, nor will we ever, because even after all that has transpired, she now lives with her parents.

I am often asked who my role models were growing up, and the only person that ever comes to mind is Nelly. She was a rock for me and taught me how to love myself even if no one else ever did. She taught me about self-respect, discipline, and to do whatever was necessary to reach a goal.

Mema baked great biscuits and one of my favorite breakfasts as a kid was eating hot biscuits with syrup on them. The reason I loved this so much wasn't the flavor. It was more the feelings I had when I ate them because of something Nelly told me every time she was there when I was eating them.

She smiled at me and said, "Now you know why you like dem biscuits so much don't you?"

I always said because they were so good.

"No it's not. Dos biscuits remind me of you, white and fluffy, with great depth, enough for a whole meal. I'm the syrup. I always go on top to keep you safe because the syrup is dark brown and sweet, just like me"

I didn't realize how true this analogy was until I was an adult. One day I was eating biscuits and syrup and contemplating a relationship I was in, and I wondered what Nelly would do. At that moment, I looked at my plate and realized Nelly would have said, "If this person isn't covering you like that syrup, you don't need 'em in your life."

Once again, my mentor, my parent, my friend, Nelly, was right.

APPENDIX A

The Court Documents

THE CITY OF SELMA

SELMA, ALABAMA 36702-0450

FAX COVER SHEET

Attention: Grant Garris	From: Selma-Police Dept
Office location: Atlanta Ga.	Date: 2-19-07
	Office location: Selma Al

☐ Urgent   ☐ Reply ASAP   ☐ Please comment   ☐ Please review   ☐ For your information

Total pages, including cover:

Comments:

I hope this will help you. This is all that I have on this case

Records Clerk

The original document faxed over to me. On the previous page a note from Lucy was written that says, "I hope this will help you. This is all that I have on this case."

ALABAMA UNIFORM INCIDENT/OFFENSE REPORT

ACJIC - 32 Rev. 5/72

Contributor's ORI	Agency Name	Date and Time of This Report	Agency Case No.
1. 0.2.7.0.1.1.0.0	Selma Police	8 ᵐᵒ 12 ᵈᵃʸ 8⁷ ʸʳ 1000 ᵗⁱᵐᵉ	8512316031 ▮

VICTIM

1. Last Name	First	Middle		5. Address (Street-City-State)		7. Phone
Garris	Grant			▮▮ -mobile AL		

4. Employer or School	5. Occupation	6. Address (Street-City-State)
Murphy High school	Student	Mobile AL

VICTIMS	8. Armed?	9. SEX	10. RAC	11. HGT	12. WGT	13. Date of Birth	14. Relationship of Victim to Offender
DESCRIPTION	☐ Yes ☐ No	M	W	6 00	150		Age 16

EVENT

15. Type of Incident or Offense (a) ☐ Fel. (b) ☐ Mad.	16. NCIC Code	17. Type of Incident or Offense (a) ☐ Fel. (b) ☐ Misd.	18. NCIC Code
Sodomy 1ˢᵗ Degree			

19. Place of Occurrence		20. Sector Number
		1 161/15

21. Point of Entry	22. Location of Victims Property
- Selma ALA	

23. Occurred on or Between			Time					24. Lighting	26. Premise Type
Month	Day	Year		S	T	T	S	☐ 1. Natural ☐ 2. Moon ☐ 3. Artificial Ext.	☐ 1. Hwy-Str-Aly ☐ 2. Commercial
-	-1	715	various	M	W	F		☒ 4. Artificial Int. ☐ 5. Unknown	☐ 3. Svc. Sta. ☐ 4. Chn. Store
Month	Day	Year	Time	S	T	T	S	25. Weather	☒ 5. Residence ☐ 6. Bank
-	-1	810	various	M	W	F		☐ 1. Clear ☐ 2. Cloudy ☐ 3. Rain ☐ 4. Fog	☐ 7. Church ☐ 8. School
								☐ 5. Snow-Sleet ☐ 6. Hail ☐7. Unknown	☐ 9. Other

27. Method of Attack	28. Tool Used (Burglary)
Involved child in oral sex repeatedly	

29. Weapon Used	30. Description of Weapon Used
☐ 1. Fire Arm ☐ 3. Hands, Fists, etc.	
☐ 2. Knife or cutting inst. ☐ 4. Other Weapon	

31. Complainant Name (Last-First-Middle)	32. Address (Street-City-State)	33. Phone
		Panama City Fla. ▮

VEHICLE – Wanted Stolen

34. Tag No.	35. State	36. Yr.	37. Tag Color	38. V.I.N.	39. ACJIS Check
					☐ Pos. ☐ Neg.

40. Veh. Yr	41. Vehicle Make	42. Veh. Mod.	43. Style	44. Color (Top) (Bottom)	45. Additional Description

Stolen Motor Vehicle Only	46. Area Stolen	47. Ownership Verified By	48. Warrant Signed
	☐ 1. Slot ☐ 2. Res ☐ 3. Rur	☐ 1. Tag Receipt ☐ 2. Bill of Sale ☐ 3. Title	☐ Yes, No. _____ ☐ No
49. Auto Insurer Name (Company)		☐ 4. License Registration ☐ 5. Other	51. Phone
		50. Address (Street-City-State)	

Motor Vehicle Recovery Only	52. Stolen in Your Jurisdiction?	53. Recovered in Your Jurisdiction?
	☐ Yes ☐ No Where?	☐ Yes ☐ No Where?

PROPERTY DESCRIPTION

54. Qty.	55. Describe Property Stolen or Recovered (Include Make, Model, Size, Type, Serial Number, Color, etc.)	56. Value Stolen	57. Recovered Date Value

COPY JUVENILE

8523003 ▮

Continue on Back

VALUE

58. Vehicles	59. Currency, Notes, etc.	60. Jewelry and Precious metals	61. Clothing and Furs	62. Office Equipment
$	$	$	$	$
63. T.V., Radio, etc.	64. Household Goods	65. Firearms	66. Consumable Goods	67. Livestock	68. Miscellaneous
$	$	$	$	$	$

ADMIN.

69. Case Status:	70. Case Disposition:	71. Reporting Officer #1 Code	75. Entered ACJIS
☒ Pending	☐ 1. Cleared by Arrest (Def. under 18 years)	Morgan Sgt BR 067	Month Day Year Time
☐ Inactive	☐ 2. Cleared by Arrest (Def. 18 Yrs. or over)	72. Reporting Officer #2 Code	☐ Person ☐ Gun
☐ Closed	☐ 3. Exc. Cleared	73. Supv. Approval	☐ Vehicle ☐ Boat
	☐ 4. Unfounded	74. Watch Cmdr. _____	☐ Article ☐ Security

TYPE OR PRINT IN BLACK INK ONLY

226

On the previous page is the first page of the incident report. This page identifies me, my grandfather where we lived and the fact that the offense is Sodomy 1st degree. The method of attack was modified from the original incident to say "involved child in oral sex respectively." There are so many personal issues I have with this statement. It would not be a charge of Sodomy in the 1st degree if it were oral sex only. There were so many other things I detailed for them that have since been removed from this report.

INCIDENT/OFFENSE REPORT Continued	Date and Time of This Report		Agency Case Number
	8 19 2 4 8 5 10 8		8 3 3 6 0 3 5

76. Name (Last-First-Middle) #1 77. Address

(age 20) Greenwood , Mississippi
(age 25) Gainsville , Florida
(age 20) Ocala , Florida

92. Name (Last-First-Middle)   J.
94. SEX M 95. RAC W 96. AGE 68 97. Date of Birth

98. Address or Probable Destination · Selma AL
99. HGT Sr./lean 5'25" 101. WGT H9% 101. EYE Brn 102. HAI 103. Complexion ruddy

104. Scars, Marks, Tattoos, Rings, Watches or Jewelry   105. Clothing Worn

COPY

NARRATIVE:

Grant Garris who is now 16 years old states that since he was about 5 years old until age 11 years old his Grand-father, _____, had performed numerous acts of oral sex with him and acts of fondling his genitals when he would be visiting the suspects residence here in Selma. He states that this problem decreased after his family moved to Mobile, and stopped after an incident in which he was approached by his Grandfather at age 14. At that time there was reportedly a verbal altercation from the victim directed towards the suspect. Nothing further occured until July 4th in Gulf Shores when the suspect is allegedly reported to have attempted to force the victim to have oral sex with him. At this time the victim reported this to his father & other family members. There are reportedly other grandchildren also involved in incidents from a number of years ago. Investigation continues.

Continue in Supplement.

I hereby affirm that I have read this report and all facts, descriptions, values and other information given by me are true and correct to the best of my knowledge and belief.
Signature of Complainant

123. IF YES, DESCRIBE IN NARRATIVE OR APPROPRIATE SECTION.

	YES	NO/UNK
Was Arrest Made? How Many? ( )		
Was There a Witness to the Crime?		
Can A Suspect Be Named?		
Can A Suspect Be Located?		
Can A Suspect Be Described?		
Can A Suspect Be Identified?		
Can Subject Vehicle Be Identified?		
Is the Stolen Property Traceable?		
Is Physical Evidence Present?		
Is A Significant M.O. Present?		
Has Evidence Tech. Been Called?		

IS THERE A SIGNIFICANT REASON TO BELIEVE THAT THE CRIME MAY BE SOLVED WITH A REASONABLE AMOUNT OF INVESTIGATIVE EFFORT? ☐ Yes ☐ No

TYPE OR PRINT IN BLACK INK ONLY

The second page of the incident report again has been modified and "softened". It states: Grant Garris who is now 16 years old states that since he was about 5 years old until age 11 years old his Grandfather, [Bernard Jowers], had performed numerous acts of oral sex with him and acts of fondling his genitals [I also spelled out for them that I was tied up, raped repeatedly and held captive on several occasions] when he would be visiting the suspect's residence here in Selma. He states that this problem decreased after his family moved to Mobile and stopped after an incident in which he was approached by his Grandfather at age 14. At that time there was reportedly a verbal altercation from the victim directed towards the suspect. Nothing further occurred until July 4th in Gulf Shores when the suspect is allegedly reported to have attempted to force the victim to have oral sex with him. At this time the victim reported this to his father and other family members. There are reportedly other grandchildren also involved in incidents from a number of years ago. Investigation continues.

COPY

ACJC- 33 Rev. 9/77   **ALABAMA UNIFORM INCIDENT/OFFENSE REPORT SUPPLEMENT**

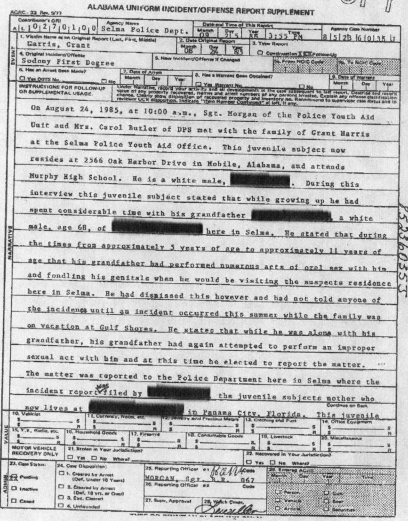

Contributor's ORI	Agency Name	Date and Time of This Report				Agency Case Number
A L 0 2 7 0 1 0 0	Selma Police Dept.	Month 08	Day 5	Year 85	3:55 PM	8 5 2 8 6 0 5 5

EVENT
1. Victim Name as on Original Report (Last, First, Middle)
Garris, Grant

2. Date Original Report — Month 08 / Day 22 / Year 85

3. Type Report — ☐ Continuation ☒ ☒ Follow-up

4. Original Incident/Offense
Sodomy First Degree

5. New Incident/Offense If Changed

5a. From NCIC Code   5b. To NCIC Code

6. Has an Arrest Been Made? ☐ Yes OBTS No. _____ ☐ No

7. Date of Arrest — Month / Day / Year

8. Has a Warrant Been Obtained? ☐ Yes Warrant No. _____ ☐ No

9. Date of Warrant — Month / Day / Year

INSTRUCTIONS FOR FOLLOW-UP OR SUPPLEMENTAL USAGE.
Under Narrative, record your activity and all developments in the case subsequent to last report. Describe and record value of any property recovered, names and arrest numbers of any persons arrested. Explain any offense classification change. Clearly show disposition of recovered property and inventory no. Recommend to supervisor case status and to reviewer UCR disposition. Indicate "Item Number Continued" at left, if any.

NARRATIVE

On August 24, 1985, at 10:00 a.m., Sgt. Morgan of the Police Youth Aid Unit and Mrs. Carol Butler of DPS met with the family of Grant Harris at the Selma Police Youth Aid Office. This juvenile subject now resides at 2566 Oak Harbor Drive in Mobile, Alabama, and attends Murphy High School. He is a white male, ▓▓▓▓▓. During this interview this juvenile subject stated that while growing up he had spent considerable time with his grandfather ▓▓▓▓▓▓▓ a white male, age 68, of ▓▓▓▓▓▓ here in Selma. He stated that during the times from approximately 5 years of age to approximately 11 years of age that his grandfather had performed numerous acts of oral sex with him and fondling his genitals when he would be visiting the suspects residence here in Selma. He had dismissed this however and had not told anyone of the incidence until an incident occurred this summer while the family was on vacation at Gulf Shores. He states that while he was alone with his grandfather, his grandfather had again attempted to perform an improper sexual act with him and at this time he elected to report the matter. The matter was reported to the Police Department here in Selma where the incident report was filed by ▓▓▓▓▓▓ the juvenile subjects mother who now lives at ▓▓▓▓▓▓ in Panama City, Florida. This juvenile

Continue on Back

VALUE

10. Vehicles	11. Currency, Notes, etc.	12. Jewelry and Precious Metals	13. Clothing and Furs	14. Office Equipment
$ ___ R	$ ___ R	$ ___ R	$ ___ R	$ ___ R
15. T.V., Radio, etc.	16. Household Goods	17. Firearms	18. Consumable Goods	19. Livestock	20. Miscellaneous
$ ___ R	$ ___ R	$ ___ R	$ ___ R	$ ___ R	$ ___ R

MOTOR VEHICLE RECOVERY ONLY
21. Stolen in Your Jurisdiction? ☐ Yes ☐ No Where?

22. Recovered in Your Jurisdiction? ☐ Yes ☐ No Where?

ADMIN

23. Case Status
☒ Pending
☐ Inactive
☐ Closed

24. Case Disposition:
☐ 1. Cleared by Arrest (Def. Under 18 Years)
☐ 2. Cleared by Arrest (Def. 18 yrs. or Over)
☐ 3. Exc. Cleared
☐ 4. Unfounded

25. Reporting Officer #1 MORGAN, Sgt. R. R.   Code 067

26. Reporting Officer #2   Code

27. Supv. Approval   28. Watch Cmdr.

29. Entered ACJIS:
Month / Day / Year / Time
☐ Person ☐ Gun
☐ Vehicle ☐ Boat
☐ Article ☐ Securities

This is the typed out version of historical incidents. This has been greatly summarized and again is very different than my testimony.

On August 24th, 1985 at 10:00 a.m. Sgt. Morgan of the Police Youth Aid Unit and Mrs. Carol Butler of DPS met with the family of Grant Harris (sic) at the Selma Police Youth Aid Office. This juvenile subject now resides at, listed is my address in Mobile, Al, and attends Murphy High School. He is a white male, DOB XX/XX/XX. During the interview this juvenile subject stated that while growing up he had spent considerable time with his Grandfather, [Bernard Jowers], a white male, age 68, of Selma Alabama. He stated that during the times from approximately 5 years of age to approximately 11 years of age that his grandfather had performed numerous acts of oral sex with him and fondling his genitals [again, omission of the rapes and beatings] when he would be visiting the suspects residence here in Selma. He had dismissed this however and had not told anyone of the incidents until an incident occurred this summer while the family was on vacation at Gulf Shores. He sates that while he was alone with his grandfather, his grandfather had again attempted to perform an improper ssexual act with him and at this time he elected to report the matter. The matter was reported to the Police Department here in Selma where the incident report was filed by the victims mother, the juvenile subjects mother who now lives in Panama City Florida.

COPY

ADDITIONAL ARREST NARRATIVE CONTINUED	Date and Time of Arrest				Agency Case Number
	Month	Day	Year	Time	8 5 2 3 6 0 3 5 J

subject is now residing with his father who lives in Mobile, Alabama. The childs mother and father are separated. It is reported that this juvenile subject had been given psychiatric care in Pensacola, Florida, and that the psychiatrist or phycologist as it maybe, in that city made the official report to the State of Alabama. Following the filing of this report the juvenile subject indicated concern that his grand-father might be involved in other juvenile subjects in the neighborhood in which he lives here in Selma. Police Youth Aid personnel and DPS personnel have made an effort to contact parents of other children in the area and have found no victims in the area and have found no other victim's or alleged victims at the time of the filing of this Supplementary Report. This juvenile's mother, however, states that she was aware that several other grandchildren in the ███ family had been victims of suspected sexual abuse by Mr. ███ also. One statement has been received by the Police Youth Aid Unit filed by ███, a female adult now living in Florida who states that she also was the victim of sexual involvement with her grandfather starring at approximately 6 years of age and ending at approximately 10 years of age. For further details regarding the juvenile subject's statement see the statement of Grant Garris and ███ incorporated into this case file. Following the filing of this report Sgt. Morgan conferred with Mr. ███ and advised him of his charges and advised him of his Miranda Rights. Sgt. Morgan was present when he was also confronted by ███, the child's mother, regarding this matter and other members of the family. Mr. ███ was advised by Sgt. Morgan that the matter would be discussed with the District Attorney's Office and either a warrant would be issued for his arrest on the above stated charge or the case would be presented to the Dallas County Grand Jury for their disposition. Mrs. Garris stated

Continue on Additional Arrest Narrative

TYPE OR PRINT IN BLACK INK ONLY

This is the second page of the type written report. It continues on describing the summary of events.

This Juvenile subject is now residing with his father who lives in Mobile, Alabama. The childs mother and father are separated. It is reported that this juvenile subject had been given psychiatric care in Pensacola, Florida, and that the psychiatrist or psychologist as it maybe, in that city made the official report to the State of Alabama. Following the filing of this report the juvenile subject indicated concern that his grandfather might be involved in other juvenile subjects in the neighborhood in which he lives here in Selma. Police Youth Aid personnel and DPS personnel have made an effort to contact parents of other children in the area and have found no victims in the area and have found no other victims or alleged victims at the time of the filing of this Supplementary Report. This juvenile's mother, however, states that she was aware that several other grandchildren in the [Jowers] family had been victims of suspected sexual abuse by Mr. [Jowers] also. One statement was received by the Police Youth Aid Unit and filed by the oldest Granddaughter of Mr. [Jowers]. **This female adult, now living in Florida, who states that she also was the victim of sexual involvement with her grandfather starting at approximately 6 years of age and ending at approximately 10 years of age. For further details regarding the juvenile subject's statement see the statement of Grant Garris and his cousin incorporated into this case file.** [These statements from me and my cousin were not part of the pages that Lucy faxed to me. Proof that further information once existed in this report that is no longer here. Two of my other cousins, who to this day can attest to this fact, also gave verbal testimony in person and that is not in my file any longer.] Following the filing of this report Sgt. Morgan conferred with Mr. [Jowers] and advised him of his charges and advised him of his Miranda Rights. Sgt. Morgan was present when he was also confronted by the child's mother regarding this matter and other members of the family. Mr. [Jowers] was advised by Sgt. Morgan that the matter would be discussed with the District Attorney's Office and either a warrant would be issued for his arrest on the above stated charge or the case would be presented to the Dallas County Grand Jury for their disposition.

COPY

ADDITIONAL ARREST NARRATIVE CONTINUED	Date and Time of Arrest				Agency Case Number
	Month	Day	Year	Time	8 5 2 3 6 0 3 5

to Sgt. Morgan that in addition to her son she felt that a total of three

other grandchildren might have been involved with their grandfather and

that she would attempt to get them to write letters to the Youth Aid

Office regarding this involvement. Only one letter has been received as of

this date, 09/25/85, that being from the above stated person ██████████

now living in Florida. ████████████ is stated as Gainesville, Florida.

This case will be presented to the Dallas County Grand Jury for

disposition as they deem appropriate. This case will be closed and

pending at this point for Grand Jury action.

Continue on Additional Arrest Narrative

TYPE OR PRINT IN BLACK INK ONLY

This is the third page of the type written report. It finishes describing the summary of events and is the very last document in my entire file. Everything else has disappeared.

Mrs. Garris stated to Sgt. Morgan that in addition to her son she felt that a total of three other grandchildren might have been involved with their grandfather and that she would attempt to get them to write letters to the Youth Aid Office regarding this involvement. Only one letter has been received as of this date 09/25/85, that being from the above stated person now living in Florida. [This was from my cousin which has obviously been removed and again, no mention of my two female cousins who gave statements in person, for a total of four victims who came forward and made official reports to the Selma Police.] This case will be presented to the Dallas County Grand Jury for disposition as thy deem appropriate. This case will be closed and pending at this point for Grand Jury action.

MYTHS ABOUT SEXUAL ABUSE/APPENDIX

There was a presentation at the fifth International Conference on Incest and Related Problems in Biel Switzerland on August 14, 1991. At this conference the National Organization on Male Sexual Victimization gave a presentation identifying seven standard myths that follow childhood sexual abuse on males.

<u>Myth #1</u> – Boys and men can't be victims.

This myth, instilled through masculine gender socialization and sometimes referred to as the "macho image," declares that males, even young boys, are not supposed to be victims or even vulnerable. We learn very early that males should be able to protect themselves. In truth, boys are children - weaker and more vulnerable than their perpetrators - who cannot really fight back. Why? The perpetrator has greater size, strength, and knowledge. This power is exercised from a position of authority, using resources such as money or other bribes, or outright threats - whatever advantage can be taken to use a child for sexual purposes.

<u>Myth #2</u> – Most sexual abuse of boys is perpetrated by homosexual males.

Pedophiles who molest boys are not expressing a homosexual orientation any more than pedophiles who molest girls are practicing heterosexual behaviors. While many child molesters have gender and/or age preferences, of those who seek out boys, the vast majority are not homosexual. They are pedophiles.

<u>Myth #3</u> – If a boy experiences sexual arousal or orgasm from abuse, this means he was a willing participant or enjoyed it.

In reality, males can respond physically to stimulation (get an erection) even in traumatic or painful sexual situations. Therapists who work with sexual offenders know that one way a perpetrator can maintain secrecy is to label the child's sexual response as an indication of his willingness to participate. "You liked it, you wanted it," they'll say.

Many survivors feel guilt and shame because they experienced physical arousal while being abused. Physical (and visual or auditory) stimulation is likely to happen in a sexual situation. It does not mean that the child wanted the experience or understood what it meant at the time.

<u>Myth #4</u> – Boys are less traumatized by the abuse experience than girls.

While some studies have found males to be less negatively affected, more studies show that long term effects are quite damaging for either sex. Males may be more damaged by society's refusal or reluctance to accept their victimization, and by their resultant belief that they must "tough it out" in silence.

<u>Myth #5</u> – Boys abused by males are or will become homosexual.

While there are different theories about how the sexual orientation develops, experts in the human sexuality field do not believe that premature sexual experiences play a significant role in late adolescent or adult sexual orientation. It is unlikely that someone can make another person a homosexual or heterosexual. Sexual orientation is a complex issue and there is no single answer or theory that explains why someone identifies himself as homosexual, heterosexual or bi-sexual. Whether perpetrated by older males or females, boys' or girls' premature sexual experiences are damaging in many ways, including confusion about one's sexual identity and orientation.

Many boys who have been abused by males erroneously believe that something about them sexually attracts males, and that this may mean they are homosexual or effeminate. Again, not true.

Pedophiles who are attracted to boys will admit that the lack of body hair and adult sexual features turns them on. The pedophile's inability to develop and maintain a healthy adult sexual relationship is the problem - not the physical features of a sexually immature boy.

<u>Myth #6</u> – The "Vampire Syndrome"—that is, boys who are sexually abused, like the victims of Count Dracula, go on to "bite" or sexually abuse others.

This myth is especially dangerous because it can create a terrible stigma for the child, that he is destined to become an offender. Boys might be treated as potential perpetrators rather than victims who need help. While it is true that most perpetrators have histories of sexual abuse, it is NOT true that most victims go on to become perpetrators.

Research by Jane Gilgun, Judith Becker and John Hunter found a primary difference between perpetrators who were sexually abused and sexually abused males who never perpetrated: non-perpetrators told about the abuse, and were believed and supported by significant people in their lives. Again, the majority of victims do not go on to become adolescent or adult perpetrators; and those who do perpetrate in adolescence usually don't perpetrate as adults if they get help when they are young.

<u>Myth #7</u> – If the perpetrator is female, the boy or adolescent should consider himself fortunate to have been initiated into heterosexual activity.

In reality, premature or coerced sex, whether by a mother, aunt, older sister, baby-sitter or other female in a position of power over a boy, causes confusion at best, and rage, depression or other problems in more negative circumstances. To be used as a sexual object by a more powerful person, male or female, is always abusive and often damaging.

Believing these myths is dangerous and damaging.

So long as society believes these myths, and teaches them to children from their earliest years, sexually abused males will be less likely to get the recognition and help they need.

As long as boys or men who have been sexually abused believe these myths, they will feel ashamed and angry.

And so long as sexually abused males believe these myths they reinforce the power of another devastating myth that all abused children struggle with: *that it was their fault.* It is never the fault of the child in a sexual situation - though perpetrators can be quite skilled at getting their victims to believe these myths and take on responsibility that is always and only their own.

For any male who has been sexually abused, becoming free of these myths is an essential part of the recovery process.

LaVergne, TN USA
10 August 2010
192740LV00003B/2/P